GODDESS

Joygopal Podder

"The fastest published Indian crime fiction author"
– LIMCA BOOK OF RECORDS

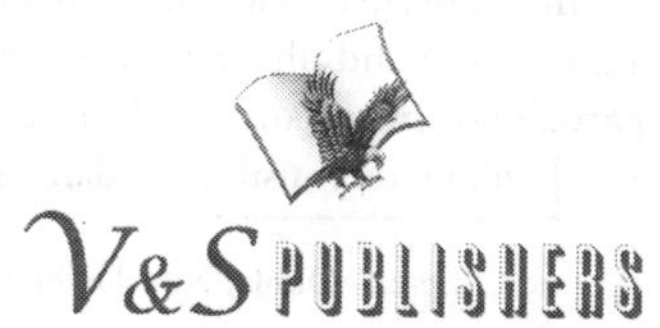

Published by:

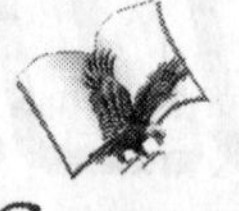

V&S PUBLISHERS

F-2/16, Ansari Road, Daryaganj, New Delhi-110002
☎ 011-23240026, 011-23240027 • *Fax:* 011-23240028
Email: info@vspublishers.com • *Website:* www.vspublishers.com

Branch : Hyderabad
5-1-707/1, Brij Bhawan (Beside Central Bank of India Lane)
Bank Street, Koti, Hyderabad - 500 095
☎ 040-24737290
E-mail: vspublishershyd@gmail.com

ISBN 978-93-505701-8-0

Edition 2013

Printed at : Param Offseters, Okhla, New Delhi-110020

Dedication

This book is dedicated to my three guiding stars – Priti, Panvi and Piya.

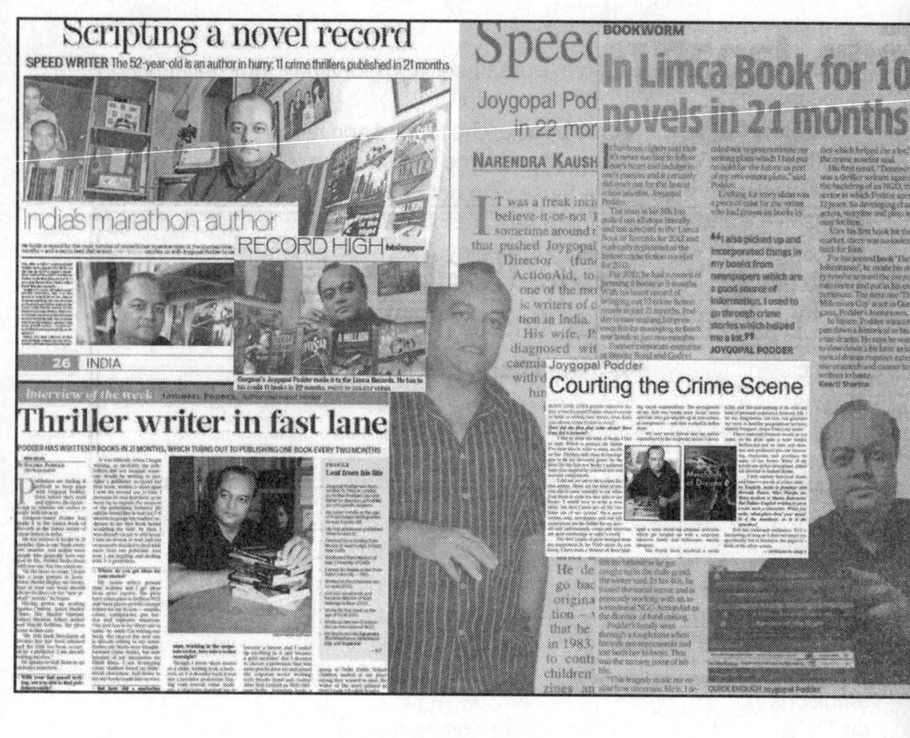

Scripting a novel record

SPEED WRITER The 52-year-old is an author in hurry: 11 crime thrillers published in 21 months

India's marathon author

RECORD HIGH

2.6 INDIA

Thriller writer in fast lane

PODDER HAS WRITTEN 11 BOOKS IN 21 MONTHS, WHICH TURNS OUT TO PUBLISHING ONE BOOK EVERY TWO MONTHS

Lead from his life

BOOKWORM

novels in 21 months

"I also picked up and incorporated things in my books from newspapers which are a good source of information. I used to go through crime stories which helped me a lot."
JOYGOPAL PODDER

Joygopal Podder

Courting the Crime Scene

Prologue

Everyone has a plan to achieve greatness and glory, until they get punched in the mouth.

This is the story of some people who tripped and fell on the slippery and obstacle filled road to greatness and fame and stardom.

This is also the story of those who got back on their feet again, dusted themselves, and carried on with fresh resolve. They went down that difficult road again – and met up with their destiny. There are others in this story that simply got screwed. I am one of those discards of fate who got buggered.

Perhaps I had it coming. Perhaps I dug my own grave. The cops and the courts certainly think so. But this really is not a story about me. I am but a side character in the drama that will unfold...

As I sit alone in my hot jail cell and stare unseeingly at the blank first page of the notebook which the prison authorities have given me in response to my application, I wonder where and how to begin the story.

Being put in solitary confinement is not something any prisoner looks forward to. It is a hellish and brutal experience, being locked up alone with yourself in a 12 x 8 feet cell. You finally understand what the word 'freedom' means in real terms. But, in my case, this forced loneliness, with all the time in the world on my hands, is also an opportunity – to pen down and relive a unique story of unique individuals, whose lives have destroyed mine...

The story I will pen is a true one; it is about two very beautiful and ambitious women. You know of them; you have read about them, seen them on TV. And I am sure most of you have seen their movies. They have risen to heights which many of you have secretly and longingly dreamt of reaching yourself. The difference between these two women and most of the rest of the world is that they went ahead and worked their butts off, and planned and schemed and got to where they wanted. The rest just dream and dream as the world passes them by.

"*Your aspirations are your possibilities,*" wrote Samuel Johnson. Rita and Sanya, from what I know about them and can guess regarding their limited literary interests, probably never read or heard this sentence – or knew of its author. But they most certainly personified this philosophy.

Those who are driven by a goal are easy to tell from those who are not. The former often have a slight faraway look in their eyes, a restlessness about them, a yearning...

You will see a lot of this restlessness in the story I will be writing. Rita and Sanya, when they entered the film industry, were both highly *driven* women. They stood apart from the crowd of star aspirants in Bollywood by their sheer focus and tunnel vision towards their goal. Their goal? They were absolutely clear about their eventual destiny – they wanted to rule the silver screen, and nobody could stand in their way. But their goals clashed. Each stood in the other's way – which was very unfortunate; which is why I am in jail.

There is this very successful Hollywood actress of several decades ago, Hedy Lamarr I think her name was, who had said: "To be a star is to own the world and all the people in it. After a taste of stardom, everything else is poverty." She was so very right. Many of the people you will meet in my story, especially the two beautiful and talented women who started off as Bollywood outsiders but went on to become screen goddesses, were touched by the terrible madness to stay on in the heavens at any cost. Their thirst for permanent glory was as boundless as the Pacific Ocean, and this led to some disastrous consequences.

Their Himalayan like ambitions made them use and discard people like children throw away once favourite toys unthinkingly but without malice, and this caused hurts which generated very unhappy repercussions...

I will dwell on some these relationships and incidents in my story. As you may, perhaps, have guessed, I am one of those who got hurt and burnt in the course of the trailblazing journey of these two divas.

It is also often not easy to carve out a new future unless you have made peace with the past. Both Rita and Sanya did stumble a bit, as many of you now know. They made mistakes. This is because they were unable to deal with the demons of their past, the immediate past in one case and the distant past in the other case – and carried these into the new and uncharted waters they chose to enter...

I really don't know why I want to write their story. Is it because my fascination for them refuses to die, irrespective of where they have brought me? Or is it because I too have many demons in my life, which I need to bury by chronicling the life story of two fascinating beauties and the way they influenced the world and the people around them? Do I need to, as the psychoanalysts say, get certain things out of my system? I don't know and I really don't care. This is a story I want to write and record. As far as I am concerned, it is as simple as that.

I have, of course, not participated in every event I will be writing so knowledgeably about, nor been privy to every conversation. But, to add on to my personal recollections of events, I also have researched a lot on the lives of the two divas from newspaper and magazine stories in the jail library while I still had a bit of freedom as an under trial prisoner. Now, of course, as a condemned convict on death row, my universe is limited to my claustrophobic cell and a bit of exercise, to the extent my injuries allow, in the jail courtyard.

Wherever I need to, I will fill in from my imagination. So some of events described may only be a dramatisation of what could actually have happened. Does it really matter? The tale of the rise of Rita Sharma and Sanya Kaushik is a gripping one, and should be told one way or the other. They shaped their own futures, while most of us allow events to shape ours. I have played a role in the drama of one of these lives; let my scenes be recorded for posterity through the pages of this book.

Drawing a deep breath I pick up the pen, bend down over the notebook, and decide to begin my narrative with my favourite person...

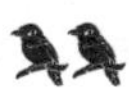

Chapter One

A STAR IS BORN

She had never ever had a feeling like this before. Not even remotely.

She was standing in front of a camera and emoting. There was a complete film crew watching her every move; she was the absolute centre of all their attention. She *commanded* their attention – and she was doing so by becoming someone else, playing another character, living another life – all for the film that was being shot, with her playing the lead role. *The lead role.*

She was the heroine of a big banner underproduction Hindi film. She was completing her first shot on the first day of the shooting schedule.

There was pin drop silence on the set as almost fifty people – spot boys, light men, make-up artists, electricians, assistant directors, production assistants, scriptwriters, cameramen and a director and a producer – listened carefully to her every word as she effortlessly uttered her well rehearsed dialogues.

It was the most dizzying, amazing, awesome experience. She felt important – *really important* – for the first time in her life.

"Cut!" yelled Dhruv Solanki – and the blinding spotlights were immediately switched off.

The camera stopped rolling. The tension on the sets eased considerably.

And then, something really amazing and stunning happened; a pair of hands clapped, then another, and then another. And then many dozens of pairs of hands joined in the chorus of clapping. The noise was quite deafening – but she felt elevated by all this sound. *They were clapping for her,* clapping thunderously as a mark of appreciation for her just concluded performance before the camera.

It was like one of those insane dreams come true.

Dhruv Solanki, the young and handsome and very demanding director of the film, wore a big smile on his face. He stepped forward and quickly planted a brief kiss on her right cheek. *In front of everybody.*

"You were brilliant!" said Dhruv, and there was a warm glow in his eyes.

Rita Sharma almost died of happiness.

Chapter Two

A PAST AND A FUTURE

Yash Kapoor stood quietly in one corner of the film set and watched the unfolding events with an impassive face.

The thrill was inside him – and a deep joy for a job well done and a gamble that had paid off.

He was happy for her. She was exactly where she wanted to be.

And she was exactly where he had wanted her to be.

He had written the dialogues which she had just spoken in front of the cameras. He had laboured long and hard over each word and each sentence. He had made the dialogues hard hitting and full of easy to understand yet brilliant nuances. Audiences would appreciate and love these dialogues – they conveyed such strength of purpose, such fire and such wit.

He had given her more smart one-liners to mouth in one film than most Bollywood actresses, even the biggest ones, got to utter in a dozen films.

He had also written the story and screenplay of this film. He had made the story completely woman oriented. The lead actress literally carried the entire film on her shoulders. It was a brilliant story, incorporating all the popular fables that had inspired generations of movie audiences the world over: an amazing journey from rags-to-riches, burning ambition, selfless and passionate love, uncompromising lovers united against an unjust and selfish world and an ending in which the weak but righteous outsmart their much stronger opponents. There was also a unique twist. The hero of the film would end up on death row. His obsession for the character played by Rita would drive him to commit murder. The climax of the film would be unexpected but eminently satisfying for all audiences and all age groups, with enough tear jerking moments to use up many thousands of handkerchiefs and many boxes of tissue paper.

The film was being made on the story he had penned not just because it was a well written one – but also because he was producing the movie. He was calling all the shots; he was the one who had put his money behind his muse, bankrolling this girl's journey to stardom and silver screen glory.

As he watched this young woman – a girl of barely twenty-one years – who he had made his protégé, walk over to her trailer for a well earned rest before the next shot, accompanied by her make-up artist, her newly appointed secretary and her elegant mother, the man smiled to himself with satisfaction. He had invested a lot of himself in this girl's potential to become a great movie star. He had his reasons for doing so, of course, a lot of them less to do with business sense and more with emotion. But his bet was likely to pay off, it appeared.

Rita Sharma was a dynamo of talent. He had been one of the first to recognise this; now others were waking up to the fact, thanks to him.

Yash Kapoor's mind went back to the evening, many months ago, when he had first seen Rita on screen. His first viewing of her on-screen persona was actually on the small screen, in an episode of a not very popular television soap in which Rita had featured in a minor role. It had been Rita Sharma's first break in Mumbai. She had appeared in only that particular episode, perhaps as a concession by the producer to the persistence of Rita's mother, whose ironclad ambition would soon become legendary. Sunita Sharma's perseverance had paid off; Rita had got a five minute role in one of the concluding episodes of the television serial.

Yash Kapoor's secretary had been badgered by Sunita Sharma to get his boss to see that episode – and assess Rita for the big screen. The secretary had been bullied – and charmed –into compliance by a fiercely determined Sunita. The producer's secretary had convinced Yash to spend five minutes watching the soap. He had actually switched on the TV set in Yash's office to ensure this.

Yash had reluctantly watched that bit of the soap, the bit which featured Rita – and had then instantly been mesmerised...

It was Rita's startling girlish beauty that had first caught his attention. But it was also more, much more. In her first scene in that episode of the TV soap, Rita had descended a staircase in the background as Poonam Khamboj, the star of the serial, stood in a drawing room setting in the foreground. Rita was a relatively tiny, unremarkable figure in the picture frame until a sudden luminous close-up took Yash Kapoor's breath away. All of his attention immediately pulled away from Poonam Khamboj, the ostensible star.

In that moment, Yash realised that Rita possessed the 'x factor' of potential stardom, what he would later refer, in many press interviews, as "the infra-red light in the dark of the movie hall".

Yash Kapoor had built his career as a celebrated film producer of Bollywood – and the careers of many aspiring actors and actresses – on the philosophy "let the camera decide". The camera had once again decided for him...

But, this time, he had been consumed by not just a desire to polish another diamond for silver screen glory. That, of course. But he had also been touched – and passionately moved – by Rita's beauty and vivacity at another level...

This was his secret.

Chapter Three

ADMIRERS

Dhruv Solanki knocked – a bit hesitantly – on the trailer door. He felt slightly unsure of himself. This was new for him – self doubt was alien to Dhruv Solanki, or had been so far...

The door of the make-up van was opened by none other than Rita's mother. She smiled at the director.

"You need Rita already? She's only been resting for ten minutes..."

Sunita Sharma was a formidable woman. She was forty-five years of age, but looked about eight or ten years younger. Her indomitable will to make her daughter into a movie star did not overshadow her impeccable charm and admirable diplomatic skills. The centre of her current universe was the producer and director of her daughter's first film. This qualified Dhruv Solanki for VIP treatment – and he got it.

"Please come in Dhruv!" said Sunita sweetly, and stepped back to allow him to enter. "I'll arrange for a beer while you wait. Rita's getting a fresh coat of make-up put on. She'll join you in a few minutes!"

Dhruv did not enter the trailer. "It's all right, Mrs. Sharma!" he responded quickly, mentally kicking himself for having come to Rita's make-up van on an impulse. "There's no need to disturb Rita. Let her take her own time to get ready. There's no hurry. The next shot is still being set up..."

Sunita looked at him speculatively. She noticed the slight unease in the young film director. "That was a brilliant shot you composed, Dhruv," she said, very quickly and smartly changing the subject in an attempt to put the director out of his obvious misery. "I'm not an expert, of course, but I was very impressed by your deft direction!"

This was Dhruv Solanki's first film as a director – and had come to him after seven years as assistant director in six films. He was pleased with all praise that came his way. He immediately warmed up to Rita's mother. "Thank you, Mrs. Sharma. Your daughter was brilliant – she gave a perfect shot!"

The mutual admiration society was disturbed by the arrival of a boy carrying a very large bouquet of flowers.

The boy, bent slightly by the burden of the gigantic bouquet, approached the trailer entrance and said: "Madam, this is for Rita ji!"

A puzzled looking Sunita Sharma picked up the card dangling from the base of the bouquet and opened it. Then a broad smiled lit up her face.

"This is from J P Mishra, the industrialist!" she exclaimed. "He saw yesterday's press conference on TV!"

The delivery boy tried not to show his impatience. "Madam, where can I put the bouquet? I will need a receipt for it, please..."

"Of course!"

As the boy left, Sunita turned back to Dhruv – and noticed that the director's face had turned serious and his forehead was creased into a frown. "Anything wrong?" she asked.

"Uh – nothing! Nothing!" Dhruv backed away and said: "I'll be waiting for Rita on the set. We'll begin shooting the scene as soon as she arrives..."

As Sunita watched the young director walk away, she realised that new challenges – as well as opportunities – had been presented to her by fate, to help her further her mission to make Rita into a big star.

Her daughter was accumulating serious admirers as she progressed. The director of her debut film was one such admirer, it appeared. And so also was the sender of the bouquet. These developments could only be for the good – if properly channelled.

Sunita Sharma once again opened the card in her hand and read the message from J P Mishra, owner of J P Industries, the third – or was it the second? – largest corporate empire of the country. *"My personal congratulations to you for your debut film, Rita. Enjoyed watching your press conference. Hope to have the pleasure of meeting you personally in the near future."*

Sunita Sharma's eyes sparkled. There was a time when doors had refused to open for her. Now, more doors were opening than she would, perhaps, be able to handle...

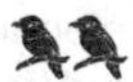

Chapter Four

THE STARMAKER

The party was in full swing. There were people everywhere, spilling out on to the first floor terrace, crowding the outdoor bar in the beautifully manicured garden, hanging out around the swimming pool. The smell of pot was heavy in the air. A skinny girl – the star of a television musical serial popular with teenagers – sat cross-legged on the floor, her thin legs pouring out of her tiny denim shorts, popping pills. A well-known Hindi-pop singer in leather trousers and matching vest snorted cocaine from a side table. Belly dancers undulated their way through the crowd, and the noise was deafening.

The noise did not disturb the host of the party, who was standing far above all the action and staring down at his happy guests from a balcony on the second floor of his palatial mansion.

The short and round man with a thick head of white hair was the most powerful movie, television and music producer in India – some sycophants said even in the whole world. This party had been thrown for his younger generation stars – the pop stars and newly minted movie and TV icons of the country. He had made them, they grew and prospered under his patronage, and no matter how crazy some of them had now become with success and drugs and the high life, they all swore unswerving loyalty and allegiance to their mentor. The great star maker Brij Bhushan Chopra...

So he rewarded them with an occasional 'no-holds-barred' party in his vast estate, as he did separately for his other more mature though not necessarily more sober stars belonging a slightly older generation. The relatively 'elder' stars partied in a different kind of an ambience – but that did not mean that debauchery in some form or the other did not grace those gatherings either.

Brij Bhushan Chopra loved pampering his stars. It kept them from straying, of course, to other predator producers and film and TV and music houses. He was vastly proud of the fact that most of the biggest stars of the country were under contract to one or the other of his companies. They were the source of his power, his prestige, his wealth.

Brij Bhushan often boasted that he "owned more stars than there were in the night sky..."

Right now, he observed from his second floor balcony perch that two of his protégés were on the verge of taking things a bit too far.

The lead actor of a new TV serial, a young hot stud with a muscular torso and tight jeans, had walked off to a corner of the terrace with the lead actress from the same show, a long haired starlet who was movie star pretty, with the requisite toned and tanned body, deep-dish cleavage exhibited in a low-cut t-shirt, and long sexy legs flowing out of a mini skirt. The young man had grabbed the girl, and pulled her in for big wet kiss. As he kissed her, his hands began exploring under the starlet's t-shirt.

The old man on the balcony raised his hand in a signal. A young man in a sober white shirt and black trousers detached himself from a group and hurried over to the passionate couple. He had seen the boss's signal; he would ensure effective disengagement, politely but firmly...

The party would not be allowed to disintegrate into an orgy – and become a source of money spinning stories for the media. Brij Bhushan's middle class audiences would tolerate only so much...

Brij Bhushan Chopra turned and re-entered his teakwood panelled study. His mind was preoccupied – and his thoughts had nothing to do with the frisky young celebrity couple whose public passion play was right now being interrupted by one of his efficient and determined executives. Nor was his mind engaged with the rollicking party he was hosting for his many young and volatile stars. Brij Bhushan strode over to his gigantic desk and once again looked at the newspapers carrying the pictures of the heartbreakingly beautiful Rita Sharma at yesterday's press conference held to announce her debut film.

How had he missed signing her up?

Chapter Five

THE DEAL

The estate was set on thirty acres of immaculately maintained parkland. It was located several miles outside the city of Mumbai, near Karjat, on the national highway to Pune. It might as well have been located in the verdant and grassy English countryside.

The surroundings were beautifully green and well populated with trees. Low capped hills contributed to the illusion that one was actually travelling through a northern Indian hill station instead of being just a couple of hours drive away from the west coast.

The estate was not just impressive – it was monstrously grand. Sunita Sharma felt a sharp fission of excitement as her car approached the heavy ornate gates.

The black Hyundai Accord was one of the perks that had come with the contract for two back-to-back movies she had signed for her daughter with Yash Kapoor. In addition to the remuneration, Yash's production company had provided the mother-daughter duo with a furnished three bedroom apartment in Juhu and a chauffeur driven car.

Sunita wondered wryly how Yash would react if he ever got to know that his car was being used to transport his new star's mother to the estate of his great Bollywood rival.

Of course, 'rival' was a wrong word to use in this context; the owner of the estate was far more powerful and successful a force to be compared in the same breath to Yash Kapoor – who was no small a Bollywood power himself. However, strong competition existed between the two – and Sunita Sharma had wisely refrained from informing either her daughter or her daughter's mentor who she was visiting this morning.

Sunita thoughtfully looked at the back of the head of her driver. His silence and confidence would need to be bought...

Sunita Sharma's thoughts were interrupted by a knocking on her car window. It was a security guard. He was dressed in a smart blue and black uniform with a peaked cap. Very impressive.

Four such guards manned the ornate gates, which were open now – but blocked by three of the men, each one holding tightly to the leash of a fierce-looking Rottweiler. The fourth guard had approached the car after it had come to a halt.

"You have an appointment, madam?" he asked very politely.

The guard was quite obviously well trained. He had no way of knowing how important this good looking and well groomed woman in the expensive car was. He knew her name, of course; it was listed in the single sheet of white paper in the slim folder he was holding. But that did not tell him her history. Given the background of the owner of the estate, this elegant woman could even be an actress – though not one the guard recognised – and could be carrying on her sensitive shoulders all the narcissism and out-of-control egomania that grew from years of public adulation. So the guard was polite, very polite, and as humble as he could be under the circumstances – without compromising on his job.

Sunita had been told the drill by the secretary of the owner of the estate. She produced her identification – her driving license. This had been scanned and e-mailed to the secretary the day before; so the guard carried the printout in his folder. He cross-checked.

Satisfied, the guard returned the license and waved the driver to enter the estate. As the car engine gunned to life again, the three Rottweilers strained at their leashes, apparently unable to bear the thought that potential prey were about to escape.

Having gained entry, the car drove up a long winding driveway, passing an elegant fountain in the forecourt, and acres of immaculately kept grounds. The house up ahead resembled a slightly smaller version of a stately European palace.

Sunita Sharma felt breathless at all the opulence. This was a lifestyle only gods could dream of! How could a mortal get so lucky!

Sunita had come to the fabled film city of Mumbai all the way from the tiny town of Dehradun at the foothills of the Himalayas, with her talented and beautiful daughter in tow, with dreams of wealth, glamour, glory and the high life in her eyes. But even she had never imagined that such riches, such power, so much grandeur could belong to one person...

The car stopped at the foot of a flight of marble steps which led to a gigantic pair of doors. A sharp looking man dressed in an equally sharp looking suit greeted her at the entrance to the house. A quick walk through a high ceilinged and thickly carpeted hallway as big as a railway station led to another flight of stairs and eventually to a teak panelled study.

Brij Bhushan Chopra got up from behind his gigantic desk and said: "Welcome, Mrs. Sharma!"

Sunita well knew the reputation of the Bollywood power she had come to meet. She was very much aware that film and television and music stars of India were born and built and died more or less at the whim of Brij Bhushan Chopra.

She knew his reputation, had heard stories of his power and his ruthlessness, and met people who feared him.

So, this ambitious mother of a talented outsider had reason to be fearful; this meeting was very important for the mother and daughter – one misstep could spell a death knell to all their dreams.

On the other hand, if all went well, who knew the heights to which Rita's career could go?

The round little man really did frighten Sunita, and as she took a seat opposite his desk, she kept her eyes fixed on him.

In spite of the full head of white hair, Brij Bhushan Chopra looked rather like a gross, thick penguin. This was widely acknowledged by all, although rarely discussed in public. The short man wore huge glasses over his eyes and had a way of looking at people that made them feel completely squashable.

Looking at him, Sunita immediately felt his vitality, but she also felt his enormous arrogance, his ego, his overbearing, driving personality. She realised that she would, perhaps, never stop being terrified of him...

But today, Brij Bhushan was very gracious.

"Thank you for coming all the way here to meet me, Mrs. Sharma!" exclaimed Brij Bhushan heartily, a broad smile lighting up his face.

*As if I had a choice...*but Sunita of course did not voice that thought.

"It is my honour and pleasure to be here, sir," responded Sunita with the right degree of humbleness in her voice.

The big man of the Indian film industry was pleased. This woman had the right attitude. He studied her – and found that he liked what he saw. There was elegance, determination, intelligence and, of course, good looks. The daughter had sprung from good genes...

"Congratulations on your daughter's debut film! The press conference of the day-before-yesterday was quite successful. There has been good coverage in the media!"

"We are blessed..."

Brij Bhushan began to eye Sunita Sharma very carefully. The woman knew how to give all the right answers...

"Yash Kapoor is a lucky man. Rita will be a great asset to his film. There's already a positive buzz about the movie! Rita is a very good actress, I have been told!"

"I hope she can live up to all the promise..."

"She will! She will! I saw her on some of the news channels, when they telecast bits of the press conference. Your daughter has an incandescent beauty. Young and innocent, with a pure virginal grace. She has a special quality, similar to a young Madhubala..." Brij Bhushan paused in the manner of an orator about to enter the meat of his speech, and then said: "But why did you not approach *me* for Rita's debut? You know, of course that I can give her a better start than anybody else in the film industry?"

This was her chance – and Sunita grabbed it with both her hands. "I did try and meet you. I tried many times! But your people did not give me any opportunity! They blocked me constantly, with all sorts of excuses!"

Brij Bhushan had heard that before – and he knew it to be a fact. He frowned to himself; the walls of protection he had created for himself worked most times; but sometimes also made him lose gems – rare gems...

"I will speak to my secretaries and managers about this. But, in the meantime, tell me: can you break your contract with Yash Kapoor?"

Sunita Sharma stiffened. "But the shooting of the film has already started! Yesterday was the first schedule! It would be highly unprofessional to attempt any such thing!"

Brij Bhushan Chopra placated the slightly agitated woman in front of him. "I do not mean that you should walk out of the first film. No, certainly not! Doing such a thing would spoil Rita's reputation at the very outset of her career – and make her many enemies, including the powerful and influential Yash Kapoor. Let Rita complete this film by all means. It will help establish her in the minds of her audiences – while she gets herself ready to stun them with her very second film, the one that *I* will produce for her!"

Sunita Sharma had the same feeling that her daughter had experienced the previous day during her inaugural shoot for her debut film. She felt like one of those insane dreams was coming true!

"You will produce a film for Rita?"

The old man nodded. "Yes I will. But first, you will have to break the two-film contract Rita has entered into with Yash Kapoor."

Sunita Sharma did not know how to react. For perhaps the first time in her life, she was stumped.

Chapter Six

THE OTHER GIRL

The Sunset View Bollywood apartments did not live up to their glamorous name. There was no sunset because they faced the wrong way, and absolutely no view. This small cluster of run-down apartments was located in a seedy side-street off Film City in Goregaon in Mumbai.

Yet the apartments were in heavy demand – from starlets and star aspirants. They were located so close to Film City, where all the action was, where work was to be found, where hopefully a glamorous future awaited...

It was late in the evening. In the sparsely and cheaply furnished drawing room of a tiny one-bedroom apartment on the second floor of one of the blocks sat a short man with deep-set hooded devil's eyes, full lips and patent-leather slicked-back hair. He wore a cobra's smile and excellent tailoring. He sat patiently, waiting. The patience paid off...

From the kitchen walked in a gorgeous beauty in tight shorts and a halter top. The shorts revealed a dangerous amount of creamy thigh. The top was cut so low that nothing much was left to the imagination. She was carrying a mug of hot coffee. The girl was a voluptuous twenty one-year-old dark haired beauty. She was perfectly lovely, except that her eyes failed to hide a maturity and world weary wisdom much beyond her years.

The girl sat down beside the short man and handed him the mug of coffee. He took a gulp of the hot liquid, put the mug on the table and slid his arm around her, pulling her in for a long kiss. After a few moments of heavy kissing activity she got to her feet, took his hand and pulled him silently into the bedroom.

Later, much later, when they were finally spent, the man lay on his back with a cigarette in his mouth and said: "I've got you a role, baby. It's a big film, with a new director and a new actress. But the hero is top rung. You'll be the second lead."

She had been stroking his bare chest with her fingers, playing with the matted hair. Now she abruptly removed her hand and raised herself on the bed, completely unconcerned that the bed sheet had fallen from her. She stared down at her lover. "Second lead? Is that all I'm good for?"

He was staring fascinated at the girl's heaving bosom. "Baby, believe me, you're better than the best! But you've got to start somewhere! The first break is always the most important! You need a good set-up for your first movie. This film has already generated a lot of buzz. It will be a sure-fire hit – and will take you to great heights along with it!"

The girl sobered down. She lay down again beside the man, but forgot to pull the bed sheet over her bare body. The man cast an admiring glance at her flat stomach and long silken legs and continued: "This is the director's debut film. He's been slogging away as a poorly paid assistant director for many years. Whenever he needed cash to maintain his high flying lifestyle, he came to me for assignments. He owes me a lot – and now it's payback time!"

The girl was not stupid. She knew she had struck lucky with this role – and that she had got it with the backing of her powerful benefactor. She leaned over and wrapped her arms around the much older man, whose cobra-like smile was now in full evidence, in obvious lustful anticipation. It was going to be a long and exciting night...

Chapter Seven

THE BILLIONARE

After J P Mishra had made his fortune and established his corporate empire, he had divorced his original wife of twenty-five years, who was not into sex any more. He had then taken on a sleek and young trophy wife number two who, after one year of marriage, conveniently forgot all the bedroom antics that had helped her snare the tycoon in the first place.

Yet J P Mishra had not discarded his second wife; she was still good arm candy and made a pretty picture with him at parties and functions. But he yearned for more. Power was the usual aphrodisiac; the richer he became the stronger became his sexual urges. His virility actually increased with age. And therein lay the seeds of his romance with the film industry...

J P Mishra financed movies so that he could mingle with stars and starlets. It was as simple as that. He had long ago learnt that sex and marriage did not jell –so he looked for the missing physical element in his life in the film studios of Mumbai.

Wealthy men do not have to hunt much for sex. If they are into paying for it – they can have as much as they want for as long as they want whenever they want. What they cannot buy, of course, is respectable sex.

At one level, Bollywood is a bargain-basement filled with second-hand talent with first-hand ambitions. Desperate starlets, all movie star pretty, with impressive cleavages and sexy legs, hosted parallel careers selling their bodies in return for much needed cash to fund their party driven lives while they waited for that one acting or item-girl break that would catapult them into silver screen glory. Tycoons like J P Mishra provided the funds they needed; the girls provided the rest...

And then the tycoon saw the newspaper pictures of Rita Sharma. He was floored. Even in a bland newspaper picture, Rita was an incandescent presence, a beauty that made men of all ages drool. She was already reputed to be a wonderful actress, too. J P Mishra wanted to own her more than he had ever wanted to own anything else in his life...

He was ready for wife number three.

Chapter Eight

ANTI-HERO

His main problem was that he had an out-of-control ego.

He was a great looking guy with a very sexy edge. Not to mention his mouth – full lips, sensual lips...lips that had many thousands of young girls drooling over his movie posters for close to two decades.

Even now, at age forty and a few months beyond, he was a teenybopper's dream – as well as fodder for the bathroom fantasies of middle-aged women. His looks, style and charisma attracted females across two generations.

But movie star glory had made him into a nightmare – insecure, narcissistic, demanding, fragile.

Shantanu Saxena had never been able to take stardom in his stride. Great fame and massive wealth had enlarged his ego to bizarre proportions. His public rantings had fed an entire industry of pulp journalists for years.

The funny thing was – the more erratic Shantanu became, the greater was his fame and notoriety, and the more valuable a property he was seen to have become in the eyes of those who financed films and made money from the Indian entertainment industry.

It would take half a dozen lifetimes for anyone to amass one million followers on twitter – and yet superstar actor, sex god, the highest paid entertainer in Indian history, playboy, alcoholic and drug abuser Shantanu Saxena had managed to achieve this feat in less than six months.

During the past half a decade, as he neared his forties, superstar Shantanu Saxena had willy-nilly re-invented himself. He had become a hot-blooded Bollywood bad boy. His television interviews were the stuff of legends. "I'm tired of pretending that I'm not special. I'm tired of pretending that I'm not a total bitching rock star from Mars!" declared Shantanu in one now very famous interview over national television a little over a year ago. In another recent interview aired on the nation's leading entertainment television channel, Shantanu declared: "I'm on a drug. It's called Shantanu Saxena. It's not available to anybody else because if you try it, you will die!"

Shantanu's newspaper and magazine interviews carried titles like: "I always win" and "I have tiger blood running through my veins".

Shantanu's over-the-top partying and many alcohol and drug binges were regular page three items in leading newspapers – often overshadowing major political dramas.

Then, six months ago, the Indian Council of Film Producers had announced that the previously declared 'Lifetime Achievement' award announced earlier in the year in favour of Shantanu Saxena had been withdrawn on grounds of his "deteriorating condition and escalating erratic conduct."

Since then, Shantanu Saxena had become one of the biggest names in the planet – his bizarre conduct faithfully followed by millions of Indians, NRIs and even non-Indians on twitter, facebook, Google, online news portals, television channels and newspapers and magazines.

What was most fascinating about the whole public drama was that, unwittingly, by his very bizarre conduct and increasing madness, Shantanu Saxena had given the world a master class in modern media promotion.

It pays to be bad – and mad. In spite of all his crazy behaviour – or because of it – Shantanu Saxena was selling more than he had ever done before...

Shantanu's last two movies, both released between four and six months ago, had gone onto become blockbuster hits.

Which explains why Yash Kapoor had buried his apprehensions and signed up the superstar to be the lead actor opposite his new find Rita Sharma.

He wanted Rita to get the best start possible, which meant ensuring that her film drew a huge initial and got packed houses on the opening weekend. There was no better way to ensure this than have Bollywood's leading superstar and most controversial actor on board the project as the film's hero.

Besides, the character to be played by the lead actor in the film demanded a touch of madness. The lead actor would be playing the character of an obsessed lover, whose tunnel vision in life focussed only on Rita's character. Shantanu possessed such obsession, he personified madness in Bollywood.

Convincing Shantanu to sign-up, however, had not been easy. "Rita *who*? Why should I act opposite a *newcomer*? Why can't you cast Katrina or Kareena or Sumeeta?"

It was a good question, of course. The top actresses of the day were dying to star opposite Shantanu; his films were almost guaranteed to be box office successes and hence give a big boost to the careers of their leading ladies. It also helped that he was a very good actor and an extremely sexy man...

Yash Kapoor did not waste time with marshalling arguments in favour of Rita's candidature. "Why don't you view her screen test and then decide?" he had simply suggested.

Shantanu Saxena had seen the screen test – and had been conquered.

His mouth had fallen open at the first glimpse of Rita on the screen. He had seen a beautiful young woman with long tousled dark hair and a devastating smile, wearing a leather jacket, jeans and combat boots. She shone on the screen, a brilliant presence that lit up her surroundings and touched everyone with a little bit of magic. And she was a wonderful actress, too...

After a few minutes of viewing, Shantanu had turned to Yash and asked: "When do we begin?"

Chapter Nine

HER BEGINNING

Rita Sharma did not realise that she was born for the camera until well into her first face-off with that piece of technology in a television studio in her hometown of Dehradun just one year ago.

She was in her final year of college, a well known debater with definitive opinions on just about everything. Her beauty had half the young men in town – and many of the older ones also – lusting after her in their dreams. One such young man had a father who owned the most popular local television channel. In order to further his 'friendship' with this gorgeous and talented beauty of his college, he invited her to participate in a television programme on his father's channel called 'Why I Love Dehradun'. She would have to prepare a ten minute essay on why she loved the town – and speak it out, with a bit of dramatic flair, on live television.

Rita had frankly never much noticed the boy; she had many such admirers since school and keeping track of the fans of her beauty and her brains had never been a priority. So she did not respond with much enthusiasm to the boy's idea and simply threw an offhand "I'll think about it" at him. But her mother, who had long been harbouring secret ambitions for her daughter, got to know about the offer – and quickly intervened.

"You *must* avail this opportunity to appear on TV, Rita! You're very presentable and speak well. You could make a career out of this!"

Rita had not given much thought to career moves. Young girls in small towns did not ordinarily do so. What she did know was that she had no intention of spending her youth as a housewife – so she decided to encourage her mother's talk about a career for her.

"You mean – become a journalist?"

"You have beauty *and* brains. Why not become an actress? A *film* actress?"

Rita had laughed. "I've acted in one play in school and none in college. That hardly qualifies for experience, mother!"

"To become an actress, all you need is for the cameras to love you, my darling – and you must learn to love the camera! Give it a try..."

Rita gave it a try just to please her mother.

The initial portents were not good, though they should have been.

Rita got enough support in the television studio, of course. She had been referred by the owner's son. That was reason enough for all staff to be sympathetic to the needs of this debutant and be supportive. The Producer of that particular programme had also been intuitive enough to observe the spark of future greatness in the young girl. The magnetic eyes of the twenty-year old girl had caught and held the attention of the programme Producer – and she immediately took Rita under her wing.

The Producer advised Rita how to behave in front of the camera. "It's easy. Sit still and get a fix straight into the camera. When the monitor rolls, you'll see your words come up on the teleprompter – all you have to do is read them. It'll look exactly like you're talking directly to the viewers."

They did a mock run-through. What an ordeal! Rita stumbled and stuttered her way through it, feeling like a complete fool. Later, she went into the make-up room where they proceeded to put too much blusher on her, and a deep green eye-shadow she hated.

"I can't stand all this make-up," she complained.

"TV lighting washes people out," the make-up assistant explained. "This way your features will come across.

So the hated make-up remained.

Next, the hairdresser teased and sprayed her hair. "Oh God! I look like a Barbie doll," she moaned, peering in the mirror.

"No, you do not. You look magnificent! Stop having a fit!" exclaimed the unsympathetic hairdresser.

By the time Rita got back in front of the camera, she was nervous.

Really nervous.

Then, suddenly, a firmness of purpose came over her.

This was no way to go live on TV! She needed to think positive and give her best! She was not going to make a fool of herself out of nervousness – no way! She had a reputation to keep as an achiever and a doer. Above all, she couldn't let her mother down, could she?

Finally, the cameras started to roll. By the time the studio manager gave her the signal to start speaking, Rita was like a greyhound at the starting gate – ready to win.

Taking a deep breath, she began to speak.

Those ten minutes in front of the television camera – and the extremely positive feedback she and her mother got over the next few weeks from what appeared to be a quarter of the population of Dehradun – were the turning points in Rita's life. The experience had thrilled her. She had found her true vocation.

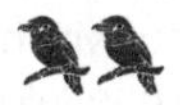

Chapter Ten

THE TRIANGLE

It was on the fifth day of the shooting schedule that Rita met her lead actor and the second lead actress.

She knew all about Shantanu Saxena, of course, and had been confused whether to thank her stars at having been gifted such a top-rung superstar hero for her first film or curse her luck at having had such a disrepute and erratic person and the acknowledged bad boy of Bollywood thrust on her.

Wisely, she had decided to keep her counsel and wait for her first meeting with Shantanu to decide whether fate had been kind or otherwise in choosing her co-star.

They met on the set. Shantanu hit the set movie star style, surrounded by an entourage. He was immediately the subject of hysterical adulation. A girl gave a small shriek and another young woman grabbed her mobile phone and started clicking pictures of the superstar. As Shantanu passed them by, film crew who were sitting got up from their chairs and stood in a show of respect. The star nodded at all of them and smiled – but did not miss a stride or stop to talk to anyone.

Rita liked her first impression of Shantanu. She had never seen any film of his, but was familiar with his handsome face through posters and television programmes. He looked even better in person. She saw an incredibly good-looking man in his late thirties with thick jet black hair, intense eyes, an athletic body and a dangerous edge.

Shantanu did not wait to be introduced to his lead actress by his director or the producer. He strode up to where Rita was sitting with her mother by her side, and smiled down at both. "Mrs. Sharma?" He looked politely at Sunita. "Rita?" he smiled. "I'm Shantanu. It's my honour and privilege to meet both of you. I've heard a lot of good things about you, Rita – and I'm looking forward to working with you..."

Both mother and daughter were floored.

The rest of the day went swimmingly. Shantanu had decided to be on his best behaviour – and it showed. He had not drunk that morning; not even beer. He had come prepared for the shoot with his lines all learnt up and rehearsed. His solo shots were all canned in one take. He behaved like a consummate professional. He was kind and courteous with Rita and her mother. He was a very helpful co-star to Rita during their scenes together, patiently giving her all the cues she needed to make her flawless dialogue deliveries, helping her with her lines – and even advising the script and dialogue writers with suggestions to improve their lines when he found Rita floundering.

All in all it was a most pleasant experience for Rita.

And then, towards the evening, Sanya Kaushik entered the set.

Sanya Kaushik was a new girl in films; that much Rita knew. Although Sanya was a movie industry newcomer, she had been personally selected for the film by the director, Dhruv Solanki. This she had come to know from her mother. Sanya was around the same age as Rita was and would be playing the third member of the love triangle also involving the film's hero and Rita's character. Hers would be a story of unrequited love; the character played by Shantanu would have no eyes for her. He would be totally smitten by Rita's character – and would go to all lengths to win her love.

Sanya was very beautiful. She had a doll-like prettiness contrasting starkly with a very sexy body. The innocence in her sweet looking face did not quite jell with her toned and tanned body, which had curves in all the right places and which was well exhibited in a tight-fitting low-cut short dress.

Sanya had come to the set dressed to seduce and kill. This put off Rita slightly – but she tried not to let any resentment show in the first meeting.

Sanya's priority, however, was not Rita. Ignoring the lead actress of the film completely, she went up to Shantanu and introduced herself. "Hi, Shantanu!" she said, extending her hand. "I'm Sanya. We'll be working together!"

Shantanu was polite; today's good behaviour would extend to everybody.

"Hi, Sanya. Glad to meet you. Look forward to working with you!" He stood up and took her hand. They had a long handshake, Rita noticed. She was sitting quietly nearby, witnessing all the drama.

Rita felt, perhaps unjustly, that Shantanu seemed quite taken by Sanya at this very first meeting. *Typical male – just because Sanya was giving him her full attention as if he was the only man on earth!*

Rita's thoughts were interrupted by Shantanu and Sanya. They had walked up to where she was sitting. "Hi, Rita," said Shantanu with a smile. "Meet Sanya, our co-star."

Rita decided to give friendship a try. She stood up and extended her hand. "Glad to meet you, Sanya," she smiled. "Hope to have many fun times together!"

Sanya smiled back, but her smile did not extend to her eyes. "I've heard a lot about you Rita," she responded, partly echoing what Shantanu had also said in the morning. They shook hands formally.

Shantanu noticed the slight tension. He wanted no part of it. "Uh, I'll leave you girls to bond; I've got to finish learning some lines..." He left.

Rita and Sanya eyed each other like wary soldiers on either side of a battlefield. "You have a shot today?" asked Rita, attempting to break the ice.

"Yes, with Shantanu. I'm trying to get across to him that I love him, but he keeps thinking only about you..."

Sanya was of course referring to the script, but there was an undercurrent in her words which Rita was not quite sure she liked.

The situation was getting uncomfortable; the moment was saved by the arrival of Dhruv Solanki.

The director was in high spirits. "Great to see you here, Sanya! Nice to find that you two have already made acquaintance! Rita's been doing a great job these last few days! The film's coming along swimmingly. Now I look forward to some great work from you, Sanya!"

Sanya grinned broadly. "I'm at your command, Dhruv! I won't let you down! Just tell me what to do." This time her smile *did* reach her eyes. As she spoke, Sanya leaned forward slightly and bent a little, so that the director couldn't miss noticing her impressive cleavage.

Rita realised that fate had delivered to her a supremely ambitious and competitive co-star, one who could, perhaps, go to all lengths to get what she wanted. But could Sanya's ambition and drive to reach the pinnacle match that of Rita's own?

Chapter Eleven

THE SECOND FILM

Brij Bhushan Chopra telephoned Sunita Sharma. This was itself a momentous act – the great film and television producer and studio owner and proprietor of music and film distribution companies did not pursue deals directly. That was a job for his managers and deal makers. But, for Rita, he followed up directly...

"Have you given a thought to my offer, Mrs. Sharma?"

Sunita Sharma gripped her mobile phone with the earnestness of one talking to divinity. "Of course I am keen that Rita's next film is produced by you, Brij Bhushan ji! But I don't want to antagonise Yash Kapoor by breaking the two-film contract mid-way through the first film. It may negatively affect his enthusiasm for Rita's debut film..."

"I understand and appreciate that, Mrs. Sharma. But do I have your assurance that Rita's next film will be with *me*?"

Sunita did not respond immediately. Frankly, the strange situation she found herself in frightened her considerably. Rita and she were new to Mumbai – in an alien land, for all practical purposes. Yash had given Rita a break after tremendous follow-up by Sunita. He had given her a powerful lead role in a high budget film. The remuneration was very good; so were the perks – the furnished apartment and the car and driver. Things were looking up; Rita was being spoken of highly and her first film was shaping up well. But all this initial euphoria had brought on many more unexpected complications.

Sunita Sharma was facing a problem of plenty. And she did not envy herself...

Left to her own devices, Sunita would have loved for Rita to work with *both* Brij Bhushan Chopra *and* Yash Kapoor. But Bollywood power dynamics and politics did not allow for that, apparently...

So how was she to answer the great Brij Bhushan?

"Rita's next film will be with you, Brij Bhushan ji," said Sunita Sharma, coming to a quick decision. "But we would still need to arrive at mutually acceptable remuneration terms and I would like to read and clear the script..."

"Of course, Mrs. Sharma! Rita's fees should not be a worry for you – she'll be paid more than what Yash Kapoor is giving. As for script – I'll put my story department to work right away to produce something powerful for your daughter..."

Sunita sat in deep thought for a long while after the phone call had ended. She had gone ahead and made a firm commitment but would now have to evaluate and then face the consequences of this assurance she had given to Brij Bhushan Chopra. She would have to break her agreement with Yash Kapoor. And she had no clue how she would do this...

Chapter Eleven

THE FIRST FILM

Well into the fourth month of the film's shooting schedule, producer Yash Kapoor and director Dhruv Solanki finally arrived at an acceptable title for Rita Sharma's debut movie, to which they both agreed and their financial backers also liked.

They called it 'Love & Death'.

The film had a unique story. Yash Kapoor had purchased the film rights of the original prize winning Hindi short story several years ago, to which he had promptly added new themes and plot twists while developing the screenplay, as befitted a Bollywood masala film. Ever since then he had been searching for the right actress to play the pivotal role in the film of the beautiful girl who inspires murder.

The original short story had been titled 'Killing for Love'. The story was that of a young man who commits murder out of love for a beautiful and idealised girl. "The kind of girl," as Yash Kapoor had explained to journalists at the press conference to announce the launch of the film with Rita in the lead role, "that a mature but romantic man gets mesmerised with on first glance and finds his eyes so fixed upon that his attention will not turn. Her beauty and poise are such that she appears to be unattainable."

Yash had gone on to add: "It might appear that Ruchita, the girl in the story, has only one responsibility that any bright, interesting and attractive girl would have in a love story, but in this case it is more – it is much more. The charisma and devastating beauty, among other attributes, of the girl Ruchita, played by Rita Sharma, is the fundamental part of the machinery that goes to make this whole story work. That is why I have waited five years to start this project; I waited five years for the right girl to come along. Rita is that girl!"

What Yash Kapoor had further explained and the journalists in attendance had faithfully reported in their write-ups was that the girl Ruchita in the film would be so compelling a character that audiences would understand – and remain sympathetic towards – the man, played by Shantanu Saxena, who had committed murder to have her.

All agreed – film industry stalwarts, the media and the public at large, after seeing her photographs in newspapers and magazines and TV grabs – that there was no better actress to create this illusion than Rita Sharma.

Some established film actresses did offer a contrary opinion, more out of envy and malice, in private and public utterances, but it did not matter; the decision had been taken.

In the months that followed the press conference, the prediction had been proven to be right. The first rushes of the film positively glowed. Even in uncut and un-dubbed freshly-shot 'raw' film that had not been enhanced in quality in film studio labs, Rita's portrayal of the idealised girl Ruchita was compelling. It was evident that audiences would understand and appreciate what drove Shantanu's character to murder; that the reasons for the man's obsession with the girl would be self-evident.

Ruchita, as played out by Rita, was staggering as far as the equilibrium of the man was concerned. And Shantanu Saxena acted out the obsessed man with a realism that came partly from his real life madness as well.

Cinematographer Mansoor Khan, whose aesthetic eye Dhruv Solanki had come to admire and trusted implicitly after seeing over and over again many of the feature films shot by him, had been instructed to shoot passively. "Use the camera to create a mood," Dhruv had told Mansoor, with a wisdom that belied his debutant director status and amazed the cinematographer. Mansoor realised that by 'creating a mood' Dhruv did not just mean capturing the play of light and shadow that so defines the visual look of a film. Rather, the director saw his camera as a "passive witness" to the beauty of his actors.

Dhruv thought that Rita's appeal was enhanced by her lack of self-consciousness, a refreshing attribute that shone through in the rushes. As the director would often state, in future press interviews, "she had this enormous beauty and she was not charmed by it." He was clearly in awe of her. He would go on to claim that Rita, in fact, "discouraged people being over impressed by her beauty."

That humility was precisely what made the character of Ruchita appealing.

Dhruv Solanki himself began to develop a unique directorial style of his own – which began to assume a kind of dictatorial shape. He began to push Rita – and everyone else – hard, very hard. One visitor to the set, a reporter from the popular film magazine 'Star and Stardust', later wrote that Dhruv drove his actors and his crew "with a sort of benign tyranny and singleness of purpose," which had the effect of uniting the cast "in the same direction and towards the same visionary goal – no mean trick in Bollywood."

Although his nature was not really autocratic – this was his first directorial assignment, after all, and he could not afford to antagonise people too much – he did not appear to much care for dissent on the sets. Certainly he got none from his young leading lady, who would go on to admit to a case of "hero worship".

The second female lead was equally cooperative. As much as she resented the importance being given to Rita in the movie and on the sets, the fiercely ambitious Sanya Kaushik learnt to hide it well. She focussed, instead, on building bridges for the future – with her talented director, who was clearly destined to make many more feature films in Bollywood. She was all cooperation on the sets, and worked really hard on her role, limited as it was. She blindly followed her director's orders, and appeared to be eager to learn from every opportunity.

Shantanu Saxena was less easy. He brooded around the set; his deep-set dark eyes seemed to burn holes in the back of Dhruv's head ever so often. Watching the director rehearse a scene with Sanya, the film's hero decided that everything was wrong. "Downbeat, blubbery, irritating" was not how Shantanu saw Sanya's character. He felt that there were better and more dignified ways of suffering in unrequited love. He loathed the way she telegraphed her "tragedy from the minute you see her on screen." She should be stronger and nobler than that, he argued. But Dhruv did not listen to him; the director had his own perspective – and he had no intention of being 'corrected' by 'ego-inflated superstars' as he once confided in private to his producer.

Shantanu also lost no opportunity to complain. "I know I'm right," Shantanu once griped to Yash Kapoor. "I'm right and I'll keep saying I'm right."

All this off-screen drama, however, did not prevent the on-screen drama from unfolding as planned. The underproduction film was soon the talk of the town; something special was being created on the sets of 'Love & Death' – and a splendid anticipation began building up among the public, partly planted by skilful pre-release promotional activity.

As the film neared completion, Yash Kapoor's publicity team got into overdrive. Rita Sharma was the focal point of the movie 'Love & Death' – and her public profile needed to be ramped up.

The first step in the strategy was to arrange for photo features in popular magazines. The media interest in Rita was high; magazines, particularly those dealing with film news and views, would welcome an opportunity to feature this beauty in their pages. Yash Kapoor's instructions to his team were simple: the photographs should be in colour, they should be full page or at least half page – and they should be such that men would not be able to turn their eyes away.

These instructions were faithfully carried out. So while Rita learnt to how to enhance her sex appeal for the movie scenes – she would, in fact, be steaming up the screen with a couple of kissing scenes with Shantanu – she also learnt how to look sultry and pose provocatively, though not indecently, for her photo features.

She developed a special rapport with the lens of a still camera. At the speed of a shutter blink, she leaped to life, displaying a verve all her own and, at the end of the process, connected magnetically with the eyes of the viewer.

Her photographers helped her to enhance her appeal in their own unique ways. "You have bosoms!" exclaimed the renowned Peter D'Costa from Goa, the photographer for the 'In Vogue' magazine photo shoot. "Stick them out!" So she did – and all around India men fell like nine pins

Chapter Twelve

TAKING CHARGE

"I want it all quick, mother! I don't want God to stop and think that I'm perhaps getting more than my share!" said Rita, after surveying the extremely positive reports about her first film in the national dailies. "When do we start the second film?"

It was Monday morning. They were sitting in Rita's bedroom. Rita was cross-legged on the bed, still in her silk pyjamas, with several newspapers and magazines strewn about her. Sunita sat on a sofa. She had woken up earlier than her daughter, and was now fully dressed for the day.

All the publications scattered on the bed carried rave reviews of the film and its lead actress. Both mother and daughter had been highly impressed with the prose used to describe Rita's performance. 'The Times of Bharat' proclaimed that Rita's "face is alive with youthful spirit, her voice has the softness of sweet song and her whole manner in this picture is one of refreshing grace." The 'Morning Star' deemed her portrayal of the beautiful girl Ruchita "one of Hindi screen's most gorgeous and magical characters so far" and the 'Uttarbharat Times' declared her "as natural and excellent an actress as you would ever hope to see."

The Friday release of 'Love & Death' had come and gone. The opening weekend had recorded brilliant collections in theatres across the country. Most movie halls had 'House Full' signs on display an hour or so before the shows began. The print and electronic media were full of rave reviews of the film and all sang praises about the performance of the three leads – Rita, Shantanu and Sanya.

During the week preceding the film's release, there had been five gala premieres and private screening events in which Rita had been the cynosure of all eyes, eclipsing even Shantanu and, of course, an increasingly disturbed Sanya. Each event had taken Rita one step closer to superstardom. The success of the film had sealed the deal.

Rita had tasted success. She loved the taste. Nothing could have been sweeter.

She also knew that she would still have been a nobody if she had not starred in 'Love & Death' – and she was therefore in a tearing hurry to begin her second film and cement her rise to superstardom.

Sunita marvelled at the change in her daughter – and felt the first signs of insecurity. How long would it be before this daughter of hers, so blessed with monstrous success, broke free?

It would be sooner than she realised...

"Brij Bhushan ji wants to sign you," she informed her daughter, a bit hesitantly.

Rita put down a magazine which carried a extremely flattering photograph of her on the cover and smiled delightedly. "That's great news mother! We can do that film as soon as I complete my second film for Yash ji! Let's try and convince Yash ji to start his film fast..."

Sunita coughed uncomfortably.

"Brij Bhushan ji does not want you to do Yash ji's second film. He wants us to break the contract."

Rita's eyes widened. "Since when does Brij Bhushan ji run our lives for us?"

Sunita's lips tightened. "Don't talk to me like that, Rita!" She softened her tone a bit. "Brij ji wants your second film to be from his stable. He feels he can give you the biggest launch vehicle of all time."

"That's very kind of him, mother. But I've already been launched. And 'Love & Death' is a super duper hit, remember?"

Sunita felt a compelling need to assert herself. "You got 'Love & Death' because of my calculated efforts – don't forget. I know what's best for you! Working with Brij ji is a heaven sent opportunity! We should not lose this chance."

"Breaking a contract with a big producer like Yash Kapoor at the beginning of my career will not be a wise thing to do, mother," responded Rita reasonably. "And Yash ji may not let me go with ease. Are we ready to fight legal cases?"

"What if Brij ji takes care of that?"

"He will still not be able to mend my reputation. Other producers will not touch me. My career will forever be hostage to Brij Bhushan Kapoor!"

Sunita accepted the strength of this argument. "Then what do we do? Annoying Brij Bhushan ji is also not such a bright idea! He'll never want to make a film with you again if you do not follow his wishes now!"

Rita looked thoughtfully at the cover photographs of herself on a couple of magazine covers and then said: "Let me speak to Brij ji."

"You think that will help? I could not convince him to let you complete the two-film contract with Yash Kapoor and *then* take on his project! You think you will be able to score where I could not?"

Rita smiled slowly. There appeared on her face a glow of self-confidence that her mother had not seen before. "I am a big star now, mother. Brij Bhushan Chopra will need me as much as I need him..."

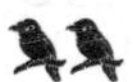

Chapter Thirteen

THE AUDITION

Sanya Kaushik had shifted out of the run-down Sunset View Bollywood apartments.

The box-office success of the film 'Love & Death' had touched all those associated with it with prosperity and good fortune. Sanya's remuneration from the movie had been quite good. She had been signed up, again as second lead, for two new projects – and had received decent advances for them. Shooting had already started for one film, and another instalment of her fee had become due. She could afford to rent a better apartment in Juhu, and buy a small car. She did both.

Her benefactor and lover, the don Raghu Basant, had taken her out for a celebratory dinner. They were eating dessert and sipping wine in the very expensive rooftop restaurant of the five star rated hotel Sea View West End.

Sanya didn't mind the expense, of course. Raghu was paying.

As usual, Raghu was nattily attired, in a smart grey jacket and light blue shirt open at the neck. The short and much older man to his girlfriend had his snake like smile plastered on his face. His deep-set hooded eyes, as usual, were fixed permanently on Sanya's bosom.

She was overflowing out of her shimmering tight-fitting low-cut short dress. Men seated at nearby tables cast covert glances in her direction. Did they recognise her from the film 'Love & Death' or were they simply attracted by the tight young body and that very pretty face?

Sanya wryly thought that it was probably the latter reason. The movie had not made her as famous as it had done Rita. Hers was not yet a well-known face. It was her physical self that was, more likely, drawing male attention her way. Men had always lusted after her – even when she had been a mere struggler.

That's how she had first met Raghu; he had saved her from one such lust driven predator...

Sanya's mind went back to that eventful day a little over one year ago, which had been about three months before she had signed up for "Love & Death" which had come to her through the efforts of Raghu Basant.

She vividly remembered the day she had first met Raghu...

Sanya had looked uncertainly out of the window as the car came to a halt in front of the building.

"This is the hotel?" she had asked the driver.

"Yes."

The building was tall and a bit imposing. There was a colourful canopy at the entrance – underneath which stood a muscular and uniformed guard. But the overall impression was not five star.

"This is not a five star hotel?" asked Sanya.

"No, its three star."

Sanya had then wrestled with her inner self, a trait she had developed when under stress. *"What shall I do? Shall I go in?"*

"You might as well go in, having come so far," replied her inner self.

The driver turned to face Sanya. "We're blocking the way," he said, his face impassive. "There are three cars waiting behind us on the driveway."

Sanya had got the hint. The uniformed guard at the entrance of the hotel had been holding the left rear door of the car open for her. She stepped out of the car.

As the Honda Civic car drove away, the driver pulled out from a pocket his cell phone while steering the car with his other hand. He pressed the speed dial button and spoke quickly to his employer. "She's in the hotel..."

Sanya Kaushik walked hesitantly up to the reception desk. A short man in a white safari suit (*"They still wear such things in Mumbai?"* wondered Sanya to herself) was standing there, talking to a black suited young man positioned behind the reception desk.

She looked from one to the other, wondering who to address her question to. She did not have to deliberate much on this, since the safari suited man spoke as she approached: "Are you Sanya Kaushik?"

Sanya was immediately at ease. She was expected. She was not amongst strangers.

"Yes, that's me."

The safari suited man, who looked like he was in his middle forties, cast an appreciative glance in her direction. Her pretty doll-like features had won his approval. "Very nice to meet you! Mr. Shakti Singh is waiting upstairs."

"Upstairs?" Sanya was surprised.

"Yes. He has reserved a suite for the audition."

The young girl swallowed. She suddenly felt very alone and very insecure. "Do auditions usually take place in hotel suites?"

The safari suited man, who had not yet introduced himself, looked stern. "Auditions, my dear girl, take place wherever it is convenient. Mr. Shakti Singh had a script reading session here this morning. He decided to carry on here for his other meetings too." The man's stern look disappeared and he attempted a smile. "The Mumbai traffic is a disaster. It's horrible at this time of the day. Doing all your meeting in one place saves a lot of time and tension."

Sanya had just been driven across half the city in Mr. Shakti Singh's car and had suffered through several traffic jams. She nodded her head vigorously, eager to show her agreement. "I understand – yes, it makes sense to do all ycur work in one place in a city like Mumbai, rather than keep moving around and get delayed..."

Sanya had reason enough to tread carefully. She certainly did not want to lose this opportunity for a role in a film, her very first. This audition opportunity had come to her after a lot of effort – she had been trying for an acting break in Hindi films for almost a year now, going from office to office, studio to studio, armed with a small portfolio of photographs and big hopes. Nothing concrete had ever materialised – only promises and "we'll get back to you" assurances. It would be silly to let her middle class inhibitions come in the way of this one big chance of a lifetime, she thought to herself.

"Shall I go up?" she asked her inner self.

"Can you afford not to?" asked her inner self in return.

"Mr. Shakti Singh is waiting." This time, there was a slight edge in the voice of the safari suited man.

"Take the risk! Go for it!" urged her inner voice.

Sanya and the man in the white safari suit entered a lift in the lobby. They stood side-by-side in the cramped space in uncomfortable silence as the lift rose to the fourth floor. Sanya felt extremely conscious in her tight fitting light pink t-shirt, which had the words 'Have A Good Day' emblazoned on the chest in green colour, and body hugging jeans. This was unusual for her. She was quite used to wearing clothes that revealed her physical attributes to best effect. But the man next to her carried an attitude that bordered almost on lecherousness. He kept casting side glances at her bosom – and God knew what else.

The lift stopped. She heaved a mental sigh of relief. They stepped out into a carpeted corridor. Sanya allowed her escort to lead the way.

The man stopped at a door and knocked. "Come in!" said a strong male voice from inside.

They went in.

The duo stepped into the drawing room of a plush suite. At one end of the room was a luxurious looking sofa set. On one side of the three seater sofa sat a familiar figure – the senior lead actor of Hindi films Shakti Singh and also the owner of this hotel. He wore a hooked nose, predator eyes, long hair tied in a pony tail, loose fitting shirt with several top buttons open and tight jeans. On the table in front of him was an open bottle of what looked like Scotch whisky and two glasses. One of the glasses was half full, the other was empty. A plate of peanuts completed the scenery on the table.

Shakti Singh was in a pleasant mood. He saw Sanya look towards the bottle of whisky on the table and said quickly: "I know, I know. It's too early in the day to start imbibing! But you how these script sessions are – so much creative thinking drains the mind and body! A little pep up is always needed after a script session – believe me, it's a professional necessity..."

Sanya had never attended a script session on her life. So she did not know what Shakti Singh was talking about. She pulled at the bottom of her t-shirt a bit self consciously and said: "How do you want me to give my audition, sir?" She looked around her. "Is there a script? Do I have to learn some lines?"

Shakti Singh looked quickly at the man in the white safari suit. "You have some other engagement, isn't it, Vinod?"

"I have, sir! Yes, I have."

The man called Vinod quickly left the room, leaving a tense Sanya eying the senior actor Shakti Singh with growing trepidation...

She again pulled at the bottom of her t-shirt and once again and looked around. The drawing room of the suite was empty but for Shakti Singh and her. "Where are the other people who will take my audition, sir?"

Shakti poured himself some whisky. "They'll be joining us shortly. But I head the panel – I decide. So, as long as I'm happy, you'll clear the audition. A fabulous movie career awaits you, my girl!"

Sanya felt slightly gratified. This sounded positive. She had struggled many months in an attempt to hear some positive comments like this...

Shakti Singh patted the sofa seat next to him. "Why are you standing like this? Come, sit!"

She crossed over to the sofa set and sat down on a single seater, ignoring Shakti's hand indicating that she join him on the three seater.

Shakti Singh looked slightly irritated at this. His took a large sip from his glass of whisky. "What's your age?" he asked.

"Twenty-one, sir!"

"That's nice and young! Ever acted in films before?"

"No, sir!"

"Commercials?"

"A couple – one chocolate ad and one short film on AIDs."

"No raunchy ads? Nothing in a swimsuit?"

Sanya looked surprised. "No, sir!"

"Why?"

This confused her. "I-I don't understand…"

The senior actor smiled benevolently at Sanya. "In films, your body is your temple. The language of cinema is spoken not just with dialogues but also with body language. In fact, the body expresses more than words ever can. If you wish to succeed in films, the last thing you can afford is inhibitions!"

Sanya was silent for a bit. She could not understand where all this was heading. She decided to change the subject – switch to a new track. "Where is the script, sir? Where are the dialogues I need to speak during the audition?"

Shakti Singh put down his glass with an air of finality. "You heard me loud and clear, my dear girl – it's your body language that will take you places more than anything else." He got to his feet. "So let me hear the language of your body!"

A cold hand clutched at Sanya's heart. She jumped to her feet. She now began to realize where all this was headed…

"I-I think I'll skip the audition today, sir!" said Sanya, edging away from the sofa.

With a swift movement, Shakti unbuttoned and then took off his shirt with a flourish. He was suddenly standing there bare-chested. "You think I've all the time in the world?" There was a rough edge in Shakti's tone. His voice was slightly harsh, his words slightly slurred. "Come! Let's stop playing games, now! You want to get into films? I'm your only chance to be a movie star! Make me happy – and you'll be made for life!" He made a move towards Sanya.

"Stop!" shouted Sanya. "I'll scream!"

Shakti's eyes blazed. "Scream all you want – this hotel belongs to me! Nobody will disturb us! Now don't make me angry. Co-operate or I'll have to use force!"

Sanya began quaking with fear. This monster was grabbing at her! She reacted instinctively. Her right hand shot up – and she planted a massive slap across the face of Shakti Singh, with a strength she never knew she possessed.

The stunned actor yelled in pain and went flying backwards. He fell in a heap on the sofa he had just vacated. There was a startled look on his face, as his left hand felt the cheek where the slap had fallen, which was then replaced by a look of great rage. *"You bitch!"* shouted Shakti Singh. "You'll pay for this!"

As Sanya looked on in horror, a knife suddenly appeared in Shakti Singh's hand. He slowly got to his feet.

Sanya should have been paralyzed with fear. She almost was. But then a wild anger began boiling up inside her – a terrible rage at her attempted exploitation. Automatically she pulled out her cell phone from her hand bag – and, in one swift motion, clicked a photo of her tormentor with the phone camera.

Shakti Singh, the ageing and very senior Hindi film actor, was caught on camera bare-chested, his eyes blazing with anger and lust and a knife in his hands…

As Shakti shouted and lunged towards her, Sanya turned and ran to the door. With shaking fingers she grabbed the door knob. She swung open the door – just as the angry man reached her. Shakti's momentum prevented him from stopping in time – his head crashed against the edge of the open door. Shakti's eyes rolled up and fell on the floor, blood gushing out from the wound on his head. His head lolled to one side. He was unconscious.

Sanya stood there for a minute, catching her breath. Shakti did not move – he lay prone on the floor.

Carefully, Sanya shut the door on the room and on Shakti. She looked up and down the corridor. There was nobody in sight. Taking a deep breath and holding carefully to her hand bag and cell phone, she walked slowly towards the lift…

Once downstairs, she quickly located the ladies restroom and gratefully took refuge inside. The restroom was empty of any other occupant. That was enough for Sanya – she broke down.

Loud sobs wracked her body for a minute and then she quietened. As she slowly recovered from the shock and horror of her recent experience, Sanya got to work repairing her face with her make-up kit. She took out her cell phone from her hand bad and ensured that the photograph of Shakti Singh had been saved. Eventually she emerged from the rest room.

There was no commotion in the lobby. Shakti Singh must have been still unconscious – or was he dead? Sanya shivered with the thought and removed it from her mind. The immediate need was to leave the hotel fast!

"Hey!" she heard a voice shout. She turned – and came face-to-face with the man in the white safari suit, the man Shakti had referred to as Vinod. He was looking strangely at her. "Everything all right?" he asked.

"No! Things are not O.K.! You're boss tried to rape me!"

Vinod turned red. "How dare you make such a wild allegation!"

"Photographs can't lie! Wait till the cops see them..."

Vinod grabbed her arm. "You're not going anywhere, you bitch! Where are the photos?"

Sanya was about to bite the hand that held her arm in a tight grip, when a cold voice said: "Leave her at once!"

Both Vinod and Sanya turned towards the direction of the voice.

The words had been uttered by a short middle-aged man with hooded eyes and slicked-back black hair. He was flanked by three tall and muscular men. All wore dark suits and black ties, like they were from some classic Hollywood Italian mafia movie or a B-grade Bollywood movie of the nineteen seventies featuring smugglers. But the short man looked genuinely dangerous. This was no cardboard cut-out of a don; here was the genuine article.

Vinod recognised the man. He quickly released Sanya from his grip.

Sanya turned and slapped the man called Vinod across his face. It was a hard slap, the noise resounding across the lobby. The youngish man behind the reception counter stared at the group with bulging eyes, but did not leave his station. He, too, had recognised the short man, it seemed.

As Vinod slowly recovered his composure, rubbing his left cheek and glaring at the young girl, the short man walked over, closely followed by his flunkies, and addressed him: "Tell Shakti to lay off this girl if he values his life." The words were spoken calmly, but carried obvious menace. "She is under my protection from now on. You know what that means, don't you?"

Vinod's face had become expressionless, but he slowly nodded his head.

The devil-eyed man then stared at Sanya and his face carried a look of unvarnished admiration. "A girl who can escape from Shakti's seduction trap in his own hotel and take his incriminating photo in the process, is special! You need have no fear of anybody in Mumbai again! I like your spunk – and I'll look after you from now on."

Sanya did not know what to make of this. Too much had happened too suddenly. Did she really need a sugar daddy? Was she stepping into another trap – from the frying pan into the fire? It would take her several weeks of wrestling with her inner self to resolve this dilemma; but the outcome was perhaps already known to her in the hidden recesses of her mind.

"No-holds-barred' ambition required patronage and backing, particularly so for a homeless expatriate in soulless Mumbai struggling on a subsistence budget and fast running out of patience, hope and stamina. It took a while, and a lot of courting by the older man, but eventually Sanya Kaushik entered into a relationship with and accepted the don Raghu Basant as her lover.

Sanya was no babe-in-the-woods. She always knew why she did what she did. She had learnt a lesson or two from her mother's life story. Sleeping with power is the closest some women can get to acquiring it themselves. And power is at a huge premium in the billion dollar film industry of Mumbai, where multi-million dollar careers are made or unmade by getting or not getting into the right movie project at the right time. Raghu would smoothen and hasten Sanya's entry into the film industry; she would make sure of that. If she offered up her body – and perhaps her heart also – to any person, it was at a price...

As for Shakti Singh? Sanya Kaushik had certainly not seen the last of him...

Chapter Fourteen
PLOTTING CAREER MOVES

The dinner date had shifted venue. The odd couple had moved to Raghu Basant's plush penthouse apartment in Bandra.

Raghu had spent lavishly at the hotel Sea View West End. He had gifted Sanya one of the best dinners in her life, replete with serenading violinists, champagne and an intimate private dining booth facing the sea.

They were celebrating the success of her first movie. She was now a star. But she was dissatisfied.

Sanya intended to convey to her powerful boyfriend that she had high expectations from him with regard to her career. She wanted to get where Rita had reached with such apparent ease – and she wanted to reach those heights fast...

As soon as she entered the extravagantly done up drawing room of Raghu's pad, Sanya flopped into a leather sofa and kicked off her shoes, wiggling her toes. Her short dress rode up to where there was no further leg to reveal, sending a rush of blood gushing into the don's head.

His eyes bulged at all that display of gleaming thigh, and he quickly walked over to the bar and poured himself a stiff shot of vodka.

Taking a gulp, he remembered to offer Sanya. "Care for a drink?"

Sanya smiled provocatively. "Of course! What about some powder to go with it?"

"I've always liked your sense of adventure, darling. Let's go for it..."

He poured her a glass of vodka, replenished his own and then opened and examined the contents of a drawer in the bar. He stepped over to where Sanya was sitting and tipped a phial of coke on to the glass-topped coffee table.

Sanya crossed her bare legs, sending a tiny shiver down Raghu's spine, took a gulp of vodka and got ready to snort some coke.

Raghu sat down beside Sanya, taking care to brush his thigh against hers, and arranged the white powder in neat lines. He then pulled out his wallet, took out a crisp five-hundred rupee note, rolled it and handed it over to Sanya.

She bent over the table, put the five hundred rupee note to her left nostril and inhaled deeply. Almost immediately she felt peaceful and powerful and sensual – all the good things.

She handed the rolled up note to Raghu, who bent and snorted some coke also. His eyes immediately glazed over.

Sanya stroked his thigh. "Darling, thanks for the wonderful evening," she said softly.

Raghu Basant smiled benignly but said nothing. He simply turned and enveloped Sanya in a tight hug. He then locked his lips in hers and launched into a long kiss, his right hand slowly and deliberately moving up her smooth as silk leg.

Later that night, before they finally made love, Sanya extracted several promises from Raghu. He would arrange finance for her next film, and produce it. He would get Dhruv Solanki who, for some reason, seemed to be unable to refuse a request from her gangster lover, to direct it. And Sanya would be this new movie's solo lead actress...

Sanya had taken another significant step towards a silver screen career which would celebrate her unbridled sexuality and which would be driven to unprecedented heights by her brazenly naked ambition.

Chapter Fifteen

THE DIVA AND THE INDUSTRIALIST

Many years ago, when J P Mishra was still building up his commercial empire, he had come into the public limelight as a result of a huge tax bill that had been slapped on him by the central government. The allegations of tax evasion had been severe; the penalty was potential imprisonment.

During that period, while his new bungalow on Delhi's prestigious Feroze Shah Road was being built, J P Mishra had lived and worked, for a few months, in a penthouse suite on the top floor of the five star Ruby Hotel on Rajpal Singh Road near the house construction site. This had made personal supervision of his dream project easy and manageable.

The unwelcome notoriety gained by J P Mishra from the income tax controversy had an unexpected repercussion – he was asked to vacate his penthouse suite by the management of Ruby Hotel.

The eviction notice was served to J P Mishra's executive assistant early in the morning. By the evening, J P Industries Limited had bought over controlling interest in the company that owned Ruby Hotel. The bait had been an outrageous premium over the existing market price of the stock – and the offer had also been coupled with a threat to go public with the unsavoury details of the wife of the hotel Chairman's on-the-sly affair with her hair stylist.

By the close of working hours of that business day, the management of Ruby Hotel had been informed by the new owners that Mr. J P Mishra would not be vacating – and that he had a list of service complaints which he wished to be addressed immediately.

Ruby Hotel was still owned by J P Industries Limited. In fact, over the years, the J P Group flagship had systematically acquired total control of the hotel's holding company, by progressively buying up shares from its owner directors and from the financial institutions and small investors who traded in it in the stock market. A final open offer was tendered to buy back the outstanding shares in the stock market at a twenty percent premium over the existing share price – and Ruby Hotel's holding company finally became a wholly owned subsidiary of J P Industries Limited. It was still one of the most profitable ventures of the J P Group.

It was in the gigantic ball room on the ground floor of this hotel that billionaire industrialist J P Mishra had organised the first ever J P Star Super Gold Awards function.

It was a grand affair.

Half of the Hindi film industry and many from the regional film industries had been flown into Delhi, at the cost of JP Industries, and accommodated in Ruby Hotel, at company expense.

The programme was a three hour long extravaganza, with many song and dance items by popular stars. J P Mishra was personally present, comfortably camped throughout the evening, except when called to present a couple of awards, in the front row of the seated audience. He was seated right next to Rita Sharma and her mother. He had quite diligently ensured that Sanya and Rita sat next to him.

The other dignitaries seated on the front row included Brij Bhushan Chopra, Yash Kapoor, Dhruv Solanki and Shantanu Saxena, amongst other stalwarts of the Indian film industry. He had greeted them all politely – but he did not appear to have much time for them after that initial exchange of pleasantries.

This was J P Mishra's first meeting with Rita Sharma. He had sent her a couple of bouquets in the past – once on the start of her first film and once when the opening weekend collections had been declared to be a record of sorts – but had never approached her for a meeting. This evening's gala was a much better way to enter her universe.

On closer inspection, J P Mishra found Rita's beauty even more mesmerising than in the photographs of her in magazines and newspapers. He had organised a private screening of her film for himself – and had been absolutely captivated. But nothing had compared to the thrill he now got – almost like that of a hot-blooded teenager with raging hormones – when he met the new superstar actress in person.

Her magnetic eyes held him in a trance. Her beauty he found absolutely mesmerising. She was also an intelligent conversationalist. They got on like a house on fire.

Thank God he had arranged for his wife to go on a holiday to Dubai with some friends of hers a couple of days before this event. She had protested – but he had got her friends to persuade her to go. If she had attended today's awards function, thought J P Mishra, she would have been like the proverbial bone in the kabab.

Sunita Sharma observed the billionaire's fascination for her daughter with mixed emotions. At one level of consciousness she was, of course, very pleased. J P Mishra had it in his power to do Rita's career a world of good. He was a film producer and financier himself – and a successful one at that, and he also had powerful connections in media and government.

But he was also a very rich and middle aged man well into his second marriage and with a playboy image. Did he have designs on Rita? That would not do, not do at all. The mother and daughter had not worked so hard to get Rita to this level of stardom to give it all up for marriage...

And did they really need another benefactor? Rita was now a star in her own right. Her problem – or rather Sunita's problem – was that of plenty; there were now too many offers and Sunita did not know how to say 'no' without causing offence. Brij Bhushan was waiting for Sanya's signal that she was ready to break Rita's contractual obligation with Yash Kapoor so that he could begin his dream project with her. Yash, of course, had no idea of this and was working hard on the script of Rita's second film project. Many other producers and directors had approached the mother-daughter duo with attractive offers, which were being considered as options after the second film was complete. If J P Mishra also had plans for a film with Rita, such a project would need to join the queue.

Times had certainly changed – for the better – for Rita and Sunita...

The award for the best debutant in a female lead role was to be announced. The anchor of the programme, the bright young hope of the movie industry, the actor Ravi Kumar, had requested debutant director Dhruv Solanki to come on stage and make the announcement of the name of the winner.

J P Mishra had not organised the awards function at great expense not to be able to have his way. This star-studded event would certainly be a marketing and branding success story – many of his products which were being promoted in the advertisement breaks during the telecast would become bigger household names – but he also had another agenda. This now unfolded.

There were four nominees. Two were from the same hit film – "Love & Death' – Rita Sharma and Sanya Kaushik.

In the sixth row from the front, a smartly dressed Sanya raised her head expectantly when her name was announced as one of the nominees for the award. She flashed a dazzling smile at the TV camera which focussed on her – and then waited with some trepidation for the winner's name to be announced.

She need not have bothered. The winner was not her. The award for the best debutant in a female lead role went to Rita Sharma.

The audience roared its approval. The clapping was thunderous.

Ravi Kumar returned to the mike, thanked Dhruv – and requested J P Mishra to present the award to Rita.

J P Mishra and Rita got up together. With a broad but dignified smile, the leading industrialist extended his hand and led a delighted looking and radiant Rita up the short flight of steps to the stage. There, he took the silver trophy in his hand from the girl attendant who had been holding it but, before presenting it to the actress, stepped up to the mike and said:

"I am honoured to have been chosen to present this special award. I truly believe that we are witness to a historic moment in the evolving journey of the Indian movie industry – the birth of a new Goddess. As Dhruv Solanki has mentioned in several press interviews and I have myself felt during the viewing of Rita Sharma's first film, she shines like an infra-red light within the darkness of a movie theatre. May her luminous presence fill our lives with joy for countless years to come..."

Then J P Mishra turned and, with a warm smile, presented an overwhelmed Rita with the trophy, as the audience once again erupted with joyful applause.

There was only one person in the audience of about a thousand who did not clap, one person whose face had twisted into a small grimace all the while J P Mishra had waxed so eloquently about Rita. No prizes for guessing – the unhappy soul was Sanya Kaushik.

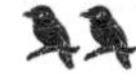

Chapter Sixteen

THE COLUMNIST

Facts were not Preetika Verma's strong point. Gossip was.

"Gossip," she had once written, in her widely read column in the film glossy 'Star Times', "has become as indispensably bound up in the making of Hindi movies as crane-mounted cameras, Swiss locales, item-songs, revenge-dramas, six-pack abs, size-zero female figures and surfboard-sized eyelashes. For Bollywood is a town doing a business based on vanity."

Preetika wrote separate gossip columns for three fortnightly film magazines and commanded more than half a million committed readers.

Her readers accepted without question every word she wrote as gospel.

Bollywood honchos and glitterati courted her, flattered her and showered her with gifts. All for a few good words in her columns. On any given day, Preetika's office or apartment would be filled with the fragrance of lilies from Kareena or lilacs from Sumeeta. Roses or boxes of chocolates from the office of Brij Bhushan Chopra were regularly delivered to her as a matter of routine; the attached cards simply read "Best Wishes". Staying on Preetika's good side was essential – because her venom was lethal.

Occasionally, well-timed tit-bits of hyped-up gossip from the pen of Preetika also helped the prospects of a soon-to-be-released film or film career. Controversy made news – and news was publicity. No news was never good news for the film fraternity, so a columnist like Preetika had assumed a very powerful position in the Bollywood landscape.

Readers lapped up Preetika's vitiol. "Bitchery," she once said, when asked to explain her success. "Sheer bitchery."

The columnist also prided herself on being ahead of events and often "creating news" and "creating news worthy stories which others picked up".

She rarely followed news and events other reporters and columnists had picked up first; once in a while, however, she found herself forced to do this.

Take the present case, for example. There was a new diva in Bollywood – and her sudden emergence had taken Preetika by surprise. This rankled. The veteran columnist had not taken very seriously the press conference that had been organised by Yash Kapoor to announce the launch of 'Love & Death'. She had not attended any of the launch events. She had been pre-occupied with other more current sensationalist stories. The film had not featured in her columns until it was half-way into its making and had already been written about by other journalists who had recognised the 'x factor' and charisma of the new lead actress and had predicted a golden future for her. Rita's rise to stardom had happened while Preetika was looking elsewhere. This slip-up was a professional disaster for the popular columnist.

After Rita had pocketed several awards and become the toast of the town, Preetika took stock of the situation – and decided to regain lost ground and take centre stage in matters pertaining to Rita Sharma.

She needed a unique story – a fresh angle to the fairy tale of the rise and rise of this new 'Goddess' as J P Mishra had referred to her at the J P Star Super Gold Awards function.

Preetika's instincts were well-honed by years as a top gossip columnist. She knew very well who would be least pleased with a lead actresses' success.

She decided to build bridges to the second lead – what was her name? Oh, yes, Sanya – Sanya Kaushik...

They met at a five star hotel coffee shop and talked over soup and salad.

They made an unlikely pair, sitting at the same restaurant table, across from each other. The columnist was short and stout, given to wearing baggy pants and loose fitting jackets. Her spectacles were designer and her hair was coiffed and she was groomed to within an inch of her life. But she was no beauty, never had been. This forty four-year-old single columnist who had remained unmarried by choice had once, over twenty five years ago, fancied for herself a career in front of the cameras. That's what she had come to Mumbai for – all the way from the sleepy central Indian town of Bhopal. From the huge windows of this top floor five star hotel coffee shop Preetika had an unobstructed view southwest over the plain of palm trees toward that glamorous area of south Mumbai where many of the film studios were located. If she squinted and imagined hard enough, she would even be able to make out Sahara Movietone Studio and Devmahal Deluxe Studio and others where she had toiled for many years as a well-dressed supporting player.

Stardom had once been a dream of Preetika's. That dream had eventually got punctured. She simply never managed to break out of the bit-parts and into the major roles. She finally had to accept the truth. She did not possess the eye-popping good looks, heart-stopping charisma, fiery talent or that indefinable 'it' that would stand her apart from the massive crowd of young women who regularly stalked the studios and producers' offices hunting for work – and stardom.

The young starlets kept getting younger, their bodies tighter – and she kept getting older.

No matter. It all eventually worked out for the best; in her case, at least, if not for other star aspirants in tinsel town. Preetika changed her calling from the film sets to the computer keyboard, first in a desperate attempt to ward off depression born of frustration and then out of a realisation that she had found her true calling.

She hated those who had raced past her to the winning post in the studios. The memories of her struggling years fuelled her vitriolic pen. She loved to dig up dirt on those who had soared up from the streets to fly in the skies; she had remained grounded, she convinced herself, so that the ballooning egos of those few who had been blessed with good genes and a few lucky breaks could be controlled – in the general interest.

Her almost missionary zeal was fuelled by the knowledge that she was now peaking in her career while those who had raced past her a decade ago were finally stumbling. She was forty-four years old, an age when most other women in Bollywood were retiring or fading into character roles and walk-on parts. But Preetika Verma was neither retiring nor fading. Rather, the industry which had once spurned her now courted her and had put her on a pedestal. She was living the best part of her life – and there seemed to be no end date in sight.

The physical contrast with the other occupant of the table was, of course, stark.

Preetika drank in the perfectly toned body with the right curves in all the right places. She liked the attitude of this girl called Sanya Kaushik. She had the best parts of her physical anatomy on show, with silken legs emerging from a short pleated skirt and, higher up, lots of cleavage show. The face was very pretty – Barbie doll pretty – but the body oozed sex. Preetika could imagine the devastating impact of such a combination on men of all ages, particularly the older ones, if projected correctly in the right kind of picture. "*What a waste she had been in a second lead role playing a tragic character burdened with unrequited love,*" thought Preetika, a sliver of an idea beginning to form at the back of her mind...

"So how has life been after "Love & Death', Sanya? Any new projects?" asked Preetika in her best interviewer style. She was friendly, eager to learn about her subject, poised to quickly pen down interesting tit-bits of information and quotes.

Sanya was still reeling from the shock of having been approached by a top columnist for an interview. *"Am I that well-known?"* wondered Sanya when she finally met up with Preetika and realised that the interview was actually going to be a reality.

Raghu Basant had advised an attitude of cautious optimism. "This woman can do wonders for our film and your career. She can make you the talk of the town, if she wants to. Tread carefully during the meeting; try and figure out what has drawn her to you."

Fighting and clawing his way up from the back lanes and chawls of Mumbai's Dharavi – Asia's largest slum – had not only toughened up the don, but had given him animal-like cunning and commonsense which Sanya had come to respect. He gave good advice to her – which she listened and followed.

"Life is good – but could be better," responded Sanya politely and with a smile.

Preetika arched her eyebrows. "Could be better? In what way?"

Sanya hesitated a bit before replying but then realised that she would be hiding nothing by not revealing the truth. "The success of 'Love & Death' has not rubbed off on all connected with the film in exactly the same way. I've signed a couple of films – but they are not starring parts."

"Not surprising, Sanya. After all, you were not the star of your first film, were you? You had a second lead role; more such will come your way. This industry is quick to cast people into stereotypes!"

Sanya smiled sweetly. "Do I look to you like a stereotype?"

Preetika began to develop a liking for this pretty, sexy, spunky girl. The tiny idea that had been germinating in her mind began to take some semblance of shape. "You don't look like a stereotype, no," responded Preetika, lying a bit. *Of course you look like a stereotype, she thought to herself – a stereotype of a flirtatious, sex-bombshell with a 'what do I care?' attitude! Baby, you've got a great future if you're packaged and marketed well!*

"But this is a tough city," Preetika continued, "and a tougher industry. Surviving in this industry is a miracle by itself. To rise above the crowd needs special talents, of course, but loads of luck – and a godfather."

Sanya coughed slightly. "I came to this city with my eyes open, Preetika ji. I know that I'll have to work hard and make a mark for myself. I have the patience – and the stamina..."

"I'm sure you have." Preetika closed her notebook firmly and put down her pen. "Look, we'll do a full interview later. Right now I want to talk to you about your career."

Sanya looked surprised. "I *have* a career..."

Preetika did not mince words. "A career like Rita Sharma's?"

Sanya bit her lips. "Not yet – but soon enough I will!"

"Only if you do the right things at the right time, have the right backing and loads of luck!"

Sanya began to feel slightly irritated. *"Why is this woman trying to put you down?"* asked her inner self. *"You don't have to tolerate her!"*

"Oh, yes I do have to listen to the likes of her!" she mentally told her inner voice. *"She's absolutely right about one thing – I do not have much of a career at the moment. What if she can help me?"*

Her inner self fell silent. So Sanya spoke: "So how do I go about getting the right kind of backing?"

"Good question! How did you land that role in Dhruv Solanki's first film?"

"I – I auditioned for it."

"Don't bullshit me, Sanya." The columnist's words were harsh but her tone was soft and she was smiling as she spoke. "You were referred into the role! How did you manage that? You surely have some kind of backing!"

"I – I have a friend."

"Who?"

Sanya debated with herself. Then she gave a mental shrug. How did it matter who knew, she decided. If her connections made her notorious – that would be news, too...

Sanya was rapidly learning the rules of the game.

"Raghu Basant."

Preetika's eyes widened. "You *do* have a smart head on your shoulders! That's serious backing – if played well."

Sanya decided that things were going too far. "Raghu is a good friend," she said firmly. "He's helped me out of several sticky situations. I respect him."

"And so you should. He gives you protection, and gets you roles in important films. What more can a girl want?"

Sanya was not sure whether Preetika meant what she was saying or was laughing at her. She decided to stand up for her lover. "Raghu is going to produce a film for me," she said proudly.

Preetika sighed inwardly. That casting couch promise again! "Sure, Sanya – but *when*?"

"He's announcing it in the trade papers this weekend. The press release and advertisement design have been sent to them. He's roping in Dhruv Solanki to direct it."

Preetika was now *very* interested. "You've got Dhruv! But he's a star director now. Hot-shot and big time! He must be costing Raghu Basant a fortune!"

"Uh – I'm not sure about the details, but Dhruv owes a lot to Raghu. He's been supported by Raghu through his struggling years. So Dhruv is obliged to Raghu and never says no to his requests..."

So that's how you got into 'Love & Death'! thought Preetika to herself, her journalistic instincts aroused like a bull at the sight of a red coloured cloth. *It'll be just fantastic to know exactly how a don like Raghu supported Dhruv in the past...*

But that would come later. Now, she had a proposition to make. Aloud she said: "Look Sanya, I think I can help you make it big in the industry – I mean really make it big!"

Sanya tried to look as if she believed her. "You will support me?"

"Big time! I really think you have that spark in you, that much talked about 'x' factor that makes stars out of ordinary people. You have oomph, sex appeal, a body to die for and a unique baby-like and innocent looking face to go with it. Cast in the right kind of project, and marketed well, you can be a bigger star than Rita Sharma!"

Sanya was sizzling from inside. She had never heard so much praise and optimism about her, and that too – to her face, ever before during her struggles in tinsel town.

Preetika was not finished. "You can project on screen what Rita Sharma, and many of the other star actresses of today, cannot. You are a sex bombshell. The others, especially Rita, have words like 'ethereal beauty, incandescent beauty and luminous beauty' used to describe them."

"How do you think I should be described?"

"With wolf whistles."

Sanya digested this. "So I should do item songs?"

Preetika smiled. "Any film you star in should be one big item song; a seducer's dance. And I have just the right script for you..."

"I think Raghu has already put a couple of writers to work on a script."

"I'm sure he has. You are a girl in a great hurry. I'm sure you would have ensured that all departments of your new film would start working overtime to put you on the screen as a leading lady as fast as possible."

"Better to be in a hurry than to be left behind," Sanya replied coolly.

"Well said. That's why you need my script. It's tailor made for you. Raghu can ask his writers to develop further my script, if they think there is room for improvement, instead of trying to write a new one. I wrote this script a couple of years ago – but couldn't think of the perfect actress to star as the seductress. I wanted a new face and now I've found the right match."

"You think Raghu will like to join hands with you?"

Preetika laughed. "Leave that to me, my girl. Your film, the kind I'm thinking of, should be big budget – much beyond what Raghu Basant can afford. It also needs enormous marketing clout. My columns will, of course, give the film huge publicity. But I can do more; I can get the biggest production house in town to partner with Raghu Basant for this film!"

Sanya stared at Preetika, her eyes round with wonder. "Which production house?"

What she heard next made her heart skip a few beats. "I'll get Brij Bhushan Chopra to back this film!" said Preetika with confidence.

Chapter Seventeen
RACE TO STARDOM

Brij Bhushan had launched into a tirade. His curses bounced off the wood panelled walls of his huge office like forcefully hit squash balls.

"That bitch! Who does she think she is?"

The two men sitting opposite him, on the other side of the pool table sized desk, squirmed uncomfortably. They were, as usual, at the receiving end of a blasting meant for somebody else.

"She's actually turned me down! *Me!*"

It was Girish Mehra who looked more upset that Rajan Pandit. After all, it was Girish who had brought the bad news.

Rita Sharma had refused to break her contract with Yash Kapoor and sign up with Brij Bhushan for her second film.

The great producer now jumped to his feet and leaned forward on his desk, placing his weight on his arms and on his hands which were flat on the table, palms down. He stared balefully at his quaking executives. He was small and he was round – but he did not look funny. His face was purple with rage. The marble eyes behind the huge glasses flashed with hatred – yes, pure unadulterated hatred. The white-haired old man was like a Roman Emperor who had been shown the finger by a child of a defeated tribe. Hundreds of heads had rolled for much less a crime. "She will pay for this! Stardom has gone to her head! I will bring her down with a thud – right back to the hard ground she belongs to..."

His executives said nothing. They were not supposed to.

The door of the office opened and Brij Bhushan's secretary of twenty years, Deepali Gadgil, walked in, carrying a tall glass of cold water in her hands.

Seeing her, Brij Bhushan calmed down a bit, but not fully. Slowly he sat down again in his leather executive chair.

The movie moghul then tore a sheet of paper from the pad in front of him, crumpled it into a tight ball – and squeezed it into the palm of his right hand with all the force he could muster, keeping his eyes closed all the while.

Slowly, the anger and tension that had built up inside him like a volcano on the boil, eased out through the clenched palm and into the crushed ball of paper.

The two executives continued to sit in silence. Deepali Gadgil held the glass of cold water tightly in her hand and waited patiently.

Brij Bhushan slowly unclenched his hand and dropped the sweat stained and crushed ball of paper on to the floor. He opened his eyes. Deepali held out the glass of water.

Brij Bhushan accepted the glass gratefully and drank the contents in one gulp.

The room heaved a collective sigh of relief. The boss was back from the brink.

The old man looked at the smartly attired young man called Girish Mehra, dressed in a starched and well ironed white shirt, jet black trousers and a sober dark blue striped tie. The frameless spectacles and well trimmed moustache gave the young man a very corporate and business-like look, the kind institutional financers and Hollywood joint venture partners of Brij Bhushan liked to see hovering around him. Girish was actually a very efficient executive – but this time had been defeated by circumstances.

"She refused to come with you?" asked the movie moghul.

Girish looked steadily back at his boss. "Yes sir. She was upset over the phone conversation you had earlier had with her."

Brij Bhushan stifled an urge to smash the glass of water against one of the walls. *"She* didn't like the way I spoke? How else was I supposed to react? That one film actress was refusing to work with me! *Me!*"

"Sir, she was refusing to break her contract with Yash Kapoor..."

"Same thing!" said the producer impatiently. "I would have taken care of any legal battle Yash would have tried to start against her! But still she refused to sign up with me. And then she backed off from her promise to meet me personally and explain herself!"

"Yes, sir. I reminded Rita that I had come to fetch her on her own request. But she told me she had changed her mind. She hadn't liked the way you spoke to her over the phone and the hurt rankled..."

Brij Bhushan shut his eyes. He was not used to this kind of treatment – and certainly not from a newcomer to the industry. What if the news spread? What would happen to the great reputation for toughness, ruthlessness and immense power that was rightfully his? Could he take this kind of challenge to his overpowering supremacy over Bollywood, lying down?

He opened his eyes and said: "I will create a star to rival this bitch Rita Sharma! I will make her a pale shadow of what she thinks she is today! *She will come to realise who makes – and breaks – stars in Bollywood!"*

There was a deep silence in the room. Girish and Rajan did not have much to say to this. Deepali debated whether to speak out what she had in her mind. The timing could not have been better. Was it destined?

Deepali was a very efficient secretary. She was more; she was also the door to the big boss. People approached her when they wanted a favour from Brij Bhushan Chopra. They ran their requests though her to gauge the kind of reaction they could expect from the big man if they were able to finally reach him. And to reach him also they needed the good offices of Deepali Gadgil. Even the powerful and feared columnist Preetika Verma.

Preetika and Deepali went back a long way. Both had come to Bollywood to become film stars, Preetika from Bhopal and Deepali from Nagpur. Both gave up the struggle – before they were forced to give up their moral scruples completely. Both took middle-class routes to salvation; Preetika took to journalism and Deepali took a secretarial course and got a job with BB Chopra Productions. She quickly caught the eye of the big man himself, and became his personal secretary.

Preetika and Deepali remained close friends. Deepali fed Preetika tips for potential scoops; Preetika kept her stories about the projects of BB Chopra Productions mostly positive – which propelled Brij Bhushan to actively encourage their friendship and treasure his secretary even more.

Brij Bhushan had jumped to his feet and was striding about the room excitedly. "Yes! Yes! That's what I'll do. I'll mentor a new star for Indian film industry! I've done it before; I'll do it again. My creation will be the new goddess of Bollywood – not Rita Sharma!"

Deepali coughed. "I may be able to recommend a newcomer with potential for this, Bhushan ji," she said.

The old man stopped in mid-stride. "Who?"

"Give me a minute, sir!" She stepped out of the room and returned almost immediately, holding a DVD cover in her hand. "I had kept this in my desk drawer, to show you sometime this week, whenever I'd find you to be relatively free. Now that the topic has come up..." She handed the DVD to her boss.

Brij Bhushan looked at it suspiciously. "What's in this?"

"It's a screen test for a new girl for a new film, the story and script of which has been written by Preetika Verma."

"Preetika writes film scripts? I thought she was completely obsessed with filling her columns with gossip and scandals. Where would she find time to write a film script?"

"Preetika wants to talk to you about her film, sir. She thinks it'll be dynamite."

"All writers think that their films will be dynamite."

"Preetika has waited years for the right actress for her script. I've seen the screen test, sir – I think this girl is special."

Brij Bhushan looked at her speculatively. "I'll have to view this DVD, of course – and give my first hand feedback to Preetika. I can't afford to antagonise your friend the columnist– her vitrol is best avoided. But I have doubts whether Preetika has managed to discover the kind of girl I want for my next film..."

He was wrong.

He got a cold chill within the first thirty seconds of viewing the DVD. Every frame radiated sex, the sensuous and limitless kind. The girl on the screen was fully clothed but oozed sex from every pore of her being. The Barbie-doll pretty girl with the soft features and red-hot body did not need a sound track; she was creating devastating effects visually.

The girl on the screen had something Brij Bhushan had not quite seen before – the capacity to be bewitching in a magnetically sexual way, not bordering on vulgar but very orgasmic all the same...

Half an hour later, Brij Bhushan had taken Preetika's telephone number from Deepali and called the columnist personally. They exchanged pleasantries. Then: "What's her name?" asked the producer.

The columnist had been expecting the call after she had got to know from her friend Deepali that Brij Bhushan had taken the DVD for a viewing. So she did not beat around the bush. "Her name's Sanya Kaushik."

"Where did you find her?"

Preetika explained the background.

"So! She was the second lead in 'Love & Death'! How interesting! That means that she will be ready to work her butt off to prove herself as a lead actress..."

"Yes, Bhushan ji. Sanya also wants to prove to the world that she can be a bigger star than Rita – who overshadowed her in 'Love & Death'!"

The old man smiled grimly to himself. That made two of them; he, too, wanted to do in Rita Sharma.

"What's your stake in all this, Preetika?"

"It's pretty simple, Bhushan ji. I want my script 'Seduction' to get made into a movie. I've waited years for the right girl – new, fresh faced, sexy and with the capacity to set men's pulses racing uncontrollably. Sanya has got that 'it' factor. She's also got a backer, who's producing and financing the film; shooting has started. But I would like a bigger banner to join in, to make the film a certifiable hit. Who but you can make 'Seduction' into the biggest movie of the Indian film industry?"

"You also want Sanya to overshadow Rita, don't you?"

"Yes. I missed the bus on Rita. She's not my story. Sanya will be *my* story – and the biggest story so far..."

"You'll promote her fully in all your columns?"

"Of course! It's *my* script that's being made into a movie, remember?"

"Who's the film's backer?"

Preetika told him.

Brij Bhushan Chopra did not like what he heard. He had scrupulously avoided any kind of contact with the underworld in all his years in the film industry. His power was so great that they had never tried to mess with him with extortion threats or strike calls. Now he would have to partner with an underworld don?

"Can't we pay off Raghu Basant and get him off the film?"

"I doubt it. He has every intention of completing the film himself. He is not averse to partnering with you to help enhance his budget and increase the prospects of the movie, this I've checked with him, but I don't think he will separate himself from the project at this stage."

"Is Sanya his girlfriend?"

"Does it matter, Bhushan ji?"

Brij Bhushan thought quickly. He had no intention of losing out on Sanya Kaushik as he had lost out on Rita Sharma. Two exciting new actresses had entered the Bollywood arena – and both were clearly destined for superstardom. At least one of them had to be from the BB Chopra stable. Otherwise, how would he be able to maintain his reputation as a star maker?

"All right," he said. "I'm in. Send me the script..."

Chapter Eighteen

A DIRECTOR IN DISTRESS

There was a crisis in the camp of Yash Kapoor. Rita Sharma's second film was ready to go on the floors, but there was no director. The director who Yash and Rita wanted on board had, to their astonishment, expressed his inability to work on the film.

Yash had been genuinely puzzled when Dhruv had told him that he would not be available for 'Story of a Superstar'. "But I had always assumed that you would direct my next film!" he told the young director, when they met up face-to-face. "It's also Rita's second film; I had taken for granted you would want to direct her again, considering the great rapport you both share."

They were sitting in the popular 'Seven Seasons' bar of a suburban five star hotel and drinking beer. Yash had requested Dhruv to join him there that afternoon, to discuss this odd situation with his protégé in pleasant and informal surroundings.

The youthful looking, tall and well built director was drawing quite a few female eyes in his direction. His face was easily recognisable, as a result of all the media interactions stemming from his recent success. He was also very good looking, in an intense and maverick kind of way, with an aquiline nose, long hair and deep set black eyes. Those eyes now looked troubled.

"Believe me, Yash, I too was looking forward to working with you and directing Rita again. She's not only a great beauty but also a gem of an actress and this movie will showcase her talents all the more. It's a great story with great potential. I would have loved to direct it."

"Then why are you not directing it?"

Dhruv took a large swallow of beer before replying. The beer gave him some strength. "My next seven-eight months are locked up in another project. I've signed another movie. It's just gone on the floors."

Yash almost dropped his beer mug. "What! That was fast! Who's the producer?"

Dhruv's discomfort was increasing by the minute. "It started off as a small project, but now it's gone big budget. Brij Bhushan Chopra has joined the project."

Yash Kapoor prided himself on his cool temperament. Nothing fazed him. This was a trait that had helped him climb the slippery ladder of success in Bollywood without too much heart burn and too much struggle. He took all challenges in his stride and moved forward regardless, without worrying too much on 'what could have been'. But this was different. This was inexplicable. His protégé was deserting his for the opposite camp! Yash felt like he had been rammed in the stomach with a sledge-hammer. It was a bit too much.

"Is it the money?" he asked quietly. "Are they paying you a fortune?"

"Uh – not exactly. No more than what you would have paid me."

"Then why, Dhruv, *why*?"

A shadow passed over the young director's eyes. But he said nothing.

Yash tried another tack. "The story attracted you?"

Dhruv nodded his head slightly. "It's an interesting story, about a young girl who's extremely sexual, very much aware of her great attractiveness to men, and who uses this strength quite intelligently to achieve power and wealth."

"A gold-digger?"

"Not exactly. It's all about a young woman in a big city without family or social support who makes her way up in life using her instincts and, of course, her sexuality."

"Sounds like a difficult role to play. Who's the actress? Can't be Rita, of course; she's tied to me for her second film."

"Brij Bhushan had wanted Rita very badly for his next film, so I have been told. But she refused to break her contract with you."

Yash looked very interested to hear this – and very gratified. "Really? I had no idea!"

"Yes. And now, a revengeful Brij Bhushan wants to create competition for Rita – so he's decided to put his weight behind this movie starring Sanya Kaushik, big time."

For the second time that afternoon, Yash almost dropped his beer mug in shock. "Sanya is starring in this movie? My second lead?"

"Yes, Yash! Sanya. You gave her the second lead role in 'Love & Death' on my recommendation, for which I'm grateful. But she wants more. And I really do believe she deserves more. You should see the initial rushes. She's lighting up the screen with her raw sexuality!"

Yash Kapoor leaned back in his chair and raised his bushy eyebrows. He stroked his neatly trimmed moustache. "You recommended Sanya for your directorial debut. Now, you're directing her first movie as a lead actress. What's going on? Are you two having an affair? Is this some casting couch kind of a deal?" he added with a slight edge in his voice.

Dhruv Solanki stiffened. He and Yash Kapoor locked stares. Dhruv was the first to avert his eyes.

"It's not what you're thinking!" said the director tightly.

"Then what is it? I gave you your big break, but since I did not tie you down to a long term contract you're deserting me at the first sign of success and running off to a competing camp! Is it for money? Is it so that you can continue f***ing some aspiring actress by godfathering her? *Why are you deserting me*?"

Yash was feeling sick to his stomach. He felt that Dhruv was being very disloyal and this betrayal was difficult for him to take in his stride.

Dhruv's eyes flashed. He leaned forward in his chair and put down his half empty mug of beer with a loud thud on the table. Fortunately, the table top was of wood, not glass, otherwise the furniture would quite likely have been destroyed. Ignoring the startled looks cast in his direction by patrons in nearby tables and passing waiters, he hissed: "I am *not* screwing Sanya. I am *not* running after money. Brij Bhushan has *not* lured me with a fortune. I still respect you and will forever be grateful for the break you gave me and the support you extended to me while our film was being made!"

"Then *why* are you doing Brij Bhushan's picture and not mine?"

Dhruv stared at his hands. "Because it's Raghu Basant's picture. He's the original producer!"

Yash continued to look aggravated. "You're confusing me! Who is Raghu Basant? Why should this person Raghu Basant make any difference?"

Dhruv's shoulders slumped a little. "I'm talking of Raghu Basant the underworld don..."

Yash Kapoor froze. His mouth fell open. He stared at the downcast face of the young man in front of him and suddenly the truth hit him with the force of a truck travelling at a hundred miles an hour. "You owe him?"

Dhruv Solanki stopped looking at his hands. He raised his eyes and returned Yash's stare. "There's no easy way to say this," said Dhruv suddenly, his body becoming very still. "So I'll try and give it to you straight." A long and silent beat. "Raghu Basant is my uncle; my mother's younger brother. I ran away from home in Ahmedabad as a teenager to join him in Mumbai and become a gangster like him. I've survived in this city because I made loads of money doing jobs for him, most of it illegal stuff. Then I fell in love with films but it took me almost a decade of struggle to become a director. The first breaks as assistant director were through my uncle's contacts. I owe him big!"

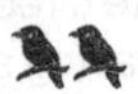

Chapter Nineteen

RIKERS ISLAND, NEW YORK

Sanya Kaushik parked her rented sports car in the parking lot of the Rikers Island prison complex in Queens in New York City. She would now have to board a private bus shuttle or a Manhattan Transport Authority bus to cross over the 1.3 kilometre Francis Buono Bridge, popularly known as the Rikers Island Bridge, which straddles the East River and is the only access to the main prison complex of New York City, housing fourteen thousand inmates, from the parking lot in the south end.

Sanya chose to board a private bus shuttle. She was soon inside the Rikers Island Visitors Centre.

The journey over the bridge had been very picturesque, but she had no eyes for it – and neither did most of the visitors to the prison complex who went there to meet an incarcerated relative or friend.

Sanya's shoulder length hair was covered by a scarf. The eyes were covered by large framed sunglasses.

The sunglasses came off at the Rikers Island Visitors Centre. They were stored in a locker along with her cellphone, hand bag and car keys. The security check was thorough, as usual. There was then the usual patient wait in the queue in the waiting area marked number 5 for the visitor pass.

This was followed by another 15 minute wait for the bus which would take her to the building in which they were holding the prisoner she had come to meet.

The bus ride was 10 minutes long. The pavements were clean and the trees were green – but the pervading atmosphere was one of greyness and gloom. There were two stops on the way at other buildings, where some of the passengers got off – on their way to meet some prison inmate or the other. Nobody went to Rikers Island to enjoy a holiday...

As she got down in front of the building which was her destination, the familiar sights greeted the young woman – but she was unmindful of them. If she had so desired she could have drunk in the not-so-distant awe-inspiring Manhattan skyline. On the left of the building entrance could be seen the La Guardia airport, where she had landed the evening before, and the Triboro and Whitestone bridges that connect Bronx, Manhattan and Queens.

Sanya ignored these phenomenal views and quickly strode into the grey building.

Inside, she went through another security check. With prior knowledge from her first visit of a couple of months before, that she would not be allowed to wear them inside the prison, Sanya had not worn any chain around her neck or any finger ring. She still had to remove her shoes and empty out her pockets – as part of a security procedure designed to prevent visitors from carrying drugs or weapons for the inmates of the jail.

This was followed by another wait.

At 3 pm they called out for her mother.

Chapter Twenty

DESIRE

Rita Sharma could not believe her ears. "Dhruv refuses to direct my next movie? Instead, he's directing Sanya Kaushik? She is his movie's heroine? He's working for Brij Bhushan ji and not you?"

Yash Kapoor drank in the look of amazement on Rita's flushed face and wondered for the umpteenth time how this beautiful girl managed to look even more gorgeous every time he saw her.

"The answer to all your questions is, yes!"

"But why?"

Yash Kapoor did not tell her. Instead, he said: "We'll get us another director, a senior player in Bollywood. How about Dheeraj Chauhan?"

Ethereal beauties do not often frown. Doing so repeatedly eventually leaves creases on the forehead, which stubbornly refuse to go away, even after the frowning stops. But Rita found herself compelled to do the unthinkable; she frowned.

"I'm sure we can get any director we want, Yash, between you and me. There's no shortage of well known people who would want to work with us, thank heaven! You have made me a big star, Yash, and I have no shortage of offers today. But I am not able to digest this rejection by Dhruv..." Her voice shook ever so slightly.

Yash had noticed the quiver in the voice and his senses went on alert. Was Rita's emotional reaction a result of professional or personal hurt?

"I will speak to Dhruv, myself!" said Rita after a brief pause. "I need an explanation."

Yash already had the explanation, straight from the horse's mouth. But could he reveal Dhruv's deep secret to Rita? The answer was, of course, no...

"Try your best, Rita," he responded, putting up a front. "But I don't think he'll change his mind. I've tried very hard with Dhruv already, as you can well believe. But he seems to have some compulsions."

"It doesn't make sense," said Rita, her lips settling into a grim line. She stood up, crossed over to the large bay windows in her living room and stared out into the deep blue ocean with half-seeing eyes.

Yash Kapoor kept sitting in the sofa and covertly studied the profile of this beautiful young woman who had come into his life not very long ago but had already made such a difference to his existence, and not just professionally. He wanted to always be around her, always make movies for her. He wanted more, much more, but there was this big problem. He was old enough to be her father.

And he was married.

He gave himself a slight shake and pulled himself together.

Rita had continued speaking.

"Dhruv is not the kind who will be bought over by money. In any case, you would not be paying him a pittance, Yash. And I know that Dhruv is comfortable working with you – and me. Besides, he also owes you an obligation; after all, you gave him his great break. How can he ditch you like this?"

Familiar words, thought Yash. *I said the very same things to him. But he is obliged to his uncle even more...*

Aloud he said: "I've given up, Rita, but that doesn't mean that *you* cannot give it a try. Speak to him yourself, certainly, if that is what you want!"

I just hope you haven't developed a very deep soft corner for him! thought Yash to himself, a bit jealously.

Sunita Sharma was not in town. She had gone back to Dehradun to settle matters with her husband, a retired army colonel now running an apple orchard. Would he now finally agree to shift to Mumbai, to be with his wife and only daughter? Or would he continue to stubbornly insist that his heart and mind would let him live only in that small town at the foothills of the Himalayas. Because then he would have to learn to live without his wife...

Sunita had no intentions of returning to her earlier ordinary middle class life in Dehradun. Not when her life's dreams were finally coming true through her daughter's brilliant silver screen career.

Rita took advantage of her mother's absence and invited Dhruv to her home for dinner. She wanted no mother around when she had her private chat with the director who she had hero-worshipped from almost the first day of shooting of 'Love & Death'. The sense of loss she had felt when Yash had told her of the director's desertion could not be explained away simply as a feeling of professional set-back. No, the feelings went much deeper. But how deep? Rita had not had occasion to examine her feelings for Dhruv in much detail till now. She had always assumed that he would be around, directing her, being an essential part of her life. But, now that this sense of permanence had been so rudely shattered, Rita felt strange emotions stir in her breast. She was suddenly enveloped by great unhappiness. She would need to deal with her feelings head on, if she did not want waves of depression to wash over her and drown her...

On the night of the dinner, Rita played the perfect hostess to Dhruv. She was constantly alert to Dhruv's every wish. Her servants were at his side the moment he finished his glass of wine, to quickly replenish it. He was kept surrounded by plates of freshly cooked delicacies and soft music soothed him as he lounged in the tastefully appointed bar lounge in Rita's apartment.

When Dhruv had entered the apartment and set eyes on Rita, he had immediately remembered his very great attraction for his film's leading lady – an attraction he had kept under control and close to his chest for fear of upsetting both their burgeoning careers.

He was again swept off his feet by her incandescent beauty, which he had so successfully captured on screen and in doing so touched the hearts of many thousands of moviegoers. He was once again captivated by her young and innocent looks, and by her sweet virginal grace.

He drank in the violet eyes, the lush black hair, the heart shaped face, the perfectly contoured body and the devastating smile...

Rita had put on minimal make-up, but had compensated with a ravishing looking low-cut dress that fell to her knees and very clearly outlined her young and beautiful body.

Rita was dressed to kill.

Rita did not come on strongly. She knew better than to do that. But she made sure that she sat close enough to Dhruv through most of the evening, and even at the dining table, so that her expensive perfume and physical and womanly charms could keep him blissfully mesmerized. Her proximity managed to move him more than she imagined; he was getting increasingly intoxicated by her closeness and dedicated attention to his needs. They made casual conversation, recalling joyous moments on the sets of 'Love & Death' and laughing over memories of funny moments while shooting.

The four glasses of red wine he had consumed before and during dinner had induced a pleasant sense of well being and peace. Dhruv was unwinding after a stressful day tying up the loose ends of his new film's script in the face of resistance from its writer Preetika Verma – and he was aware and appreciative that it was Rita's hospitality and company which was making him so comfortable and relaxed.

It was long after dinner. The servants had retired to other corners of the large apartment. Dhruv was sitting contentedly next to Rita in a comfortable sofa facing her favourite bay windows. The windows offered a clear view of the night time sea sprinkled with stray lights from faraway ships in anchor. Rita turned her face slightly and stared intently at the young director.

"I'm looking forward to working with you in my next film, Dhruv," she said a bit abruptly, unable to hold back any longer. "You understood me perfectly when we worked on 'Love & Death'. I need a strong and sensitive director like you to bring out the best in me. I can't think of anybody else directing me."

Dhruv went still. In spite of himself, he began to feel the familiar wave of helplessness creep up on him. The feeling had been on the ascendency recently, this bitterness at not being master of his own destiny. How long would he have to be obliged to his uncle for his past support? When would his choices be his alone, uninfluenced by the dictates and agendas of others?

Rita did not wait for a reaction. She continued: "When Yash presented me with the script of 'Story of a Superstar', he had told me that he would ask you to direct it. I was very happy to know this and studied the script with great enthusiasm. After reading it, I was even more convinced that it would be an ideal film for you to direct. I identified with the character of the innocent yet ambitious girl in the story who accidentally trips into stardom, and her loves and tragedies, because I knew you would be guiding me through the role. You're doing this project, aren't you?"

Dhruv felt as if walls were closing in on him, but he fought back. He looked straight into Rita's deep violet eyes. "Yash told you that I had declined to work in this film, isn't it? You're trying to make me change my mind?"

Rita did not pull her eyes away. She did not want to. Dhruv Solanki touched her where she had never been touched before. She no longer saw just an intense director; she saw more. She saw a good-looking young man with liquid eyes and a sensitive face. She loved the way his hair fell on his forehead, and his body was –

She pulled herself together.

"So what if I *am* trying to change your mind, Dhruv?" replied Rita, throwing caution to the winds. "Why should I not want you to direct me? You and I have a very special connection. Will you deny that?"

There was a strong moment of silence between them. Then Dhruv got to his feet abruptly, and the moment passed. "I've committed myself to my uncle's film!" he said roughly. "I can't back out."

Rita also got to her feet. "Your uncle, Dhruv? Who are you referring to?"

Dhruv realised with a shock that the combination of wine and Rita's closeness and persistence – and his own feeling of helplessness, perhaps – had made him reveal more than he had intended to.

"Can you keep this to yourself, Rita?" he asked, once again looking straight at her with his strangely intense yet vulnerable eyes.

Two things happened. Rita drowned in those intense eyes and she felt a wave of desire that almost choked her.

"Tell me what's troubling you, Dhruv," she said softly, after controlling her emotions with some difficulty. "What you tell me will remain with me only..."

There was another long silent moment as their eyes met. Dhruv melted irrevocably. He reached out and took her hand and sat her down back on the sofa. He sat down beside her. He told her about his obligations to Raghu Basant. He spoke of his difficult initial years in Mumbai, about his work for his uncle, the extortions, the drug dealing, the break-ins. He spoke of his struggles to become a director, of the early breaks he had got because of his uncle's contacts.

Rita was shocked but not revolted. She had seen, experienced and profited from this gifted director's immense talent. She admired the manner in which he had broken out from his initial destiny and had carved out a new one – a brilliant one – for himself.

Rita raised her right hand and placed it on Dhruv's cheek. "I understand now, Dhruv, and I can feel your pain, your conflict, your dilemma. I don't envy you the pressure you're under. I am with you in your struggle; we'll find a way out..."

Their eyes locked. They both knew that they were on a collision course and neither wished to stop the inevitable.

Rita felt like she had been jolted with a shot of electricity. Dhruv's eyes were so impossibly black and silken. His features shone with such sensitivity. She raised her lips and planted them full on his. He reached out and held her. They kissed, long and passionately.

A little later that night, they made love. Their love making was gentle. They let the climax build slowly until the pent up desires could be held back no more. The journey to blissful ecstasy was then short and swift, leaving them joyous and deeply enveloped in glorious love.

Chapter Twenty-One

A SUPERSTAR STRIKES BACK

Nobody can be more vengeful than an egocentric jerk.

Shantanu Saxena was a superstar. So he had a super sized ego. It came with the territory.

For all the years he had been a superstar, he had only thought of what he had wanted and damn the rest of the world. It had always been me, me, and me. *My* life, *my* looks, *my* career, *my* likes.

So it had been very difficult to stomach the fact that, on the sets of 'Love and Death', it was her director and not her lead actor that Rita had been singularly drawn to.

Shantanu had made that out clearly. He was not blind.

The other actress – what was her name? – yes, Sanya, was all over him on the sets, on the few occasions they shot together. But Sanya did not interest Shantanu. Rita did.

Rita was the reason he had signed on for the film, in the first place.

The first glimpse that Shantanu had got of Rita on the screen, when he had viewed her screen test on the insistence of Yash Kapoor, had electrified him. He had been touched by her magic in more ways than one. They got close, obviously, while shooting for the movie, and he could see that she liked him. He had been on his best behaviour throughout the film shooting schedule, so that he could impress her, which he did, he knew, but it never developed beyond that.

They had shared two kisses for the film. He had greatly enjoyed kissing her. But they had been single take shots; there had been no opportunity to prolong those golden opportunities.

Rita had kissable lips; Shantanu had enjoyed locking his lips with them. But a film kiss is a professional one; there is no room for dragging the lip locks beyond the dictates of the specific screen time allotted. There are film crew members observing every move – cameramen, light men, sound recordists, and the mother of the actress and, of course, the director himself. Hardly an environment to encourage the birth of passionate feelings between the kissers.

No, Rita had not fallen for Shantanu, in spite of his wishes and efforts. That was a shock. A bigger shock was that she appeared to have chosen Dhruv over him when it came to having a soft corner for anybody. Her eyes would literally gleam in Dhruv's presence. She hero-worshipped him. This was difficult to digest by Shantanu the superstar.

Why had this happened? Was it because Dhruv was much younger than Shantanu, and closer to Rita's age? Was it because Dhruv, being the director, wielded visible power and authority on the sets? Was Shantanu's superstar status – and his looks and fame and wealth – of no consequence?

The movie had come and gone without any progress made by Shantanu in the direction of wining Rita's heart. That was a personal setback. There was also a professional piece of bad news. All credit for the movie's grand success had gone to Rita and Dhruv. He didn't figure much in the accolades.

The rave reviews had been for the lead actress and director. The media which had gone ga-ga over 'Love & Death' had extensively interviewed Rita and Dhruv. There were also occasional interviews done of Shantanu and Sanya, but nowhere near the volume notched up by Rita and Dhruv. It was not a numbers game – it was a reflection of popularity and mass adulation. Shantanu Saxena had slipped – rapidly overtaken by the newcomer actress Rita Sharma and also by the debutant director of the film Dhruv Solanki.

The superstar's super sized ego wanted revenge. Badly.

He brooded over booze. He brooded more while high on dope. And slowly several plans began to take shape.

He would knock Rita and Dhruv off their recently acquired pedestals.

He would sabotage their careers.

He would eventually bed a remorseful Rita.

Nothing could penetrate that gigantic and out-of-control ego to alert the erratic and narcissistic superstar that his dreams of playing God were a bit farfetched...

After deep thought, Shantanu telephoned Brij Bhushan Chopra. "I want to make a film with you, Brij ji. I will partly finance it."

Brij Bhushan had taken the call immediately since he had recognised the number stored in his mobile phone memory. He and Shantanu did not talk often now, but there had been a time when they had been very close.

Shantanu Saxena had been a discovery of Brij Bhushan Chopra's late son.

Shantanu had been a mere boy of twenty or twenty one years, a struggler in the Hindi movie industry and an outsider with no contacts or patrons, when the twenty five year old son of Brij Bhushan Chopra had spotted him in a film party, two decades ago. Brij Bhushan's son had just then, a year or so back, after graduating from the US, joined his father's rapidly growing entertainment empire – and was eager to make a mark.

He felt that Shantanu had a certain spark; he felt that the young actor who had till then done just a couple of bit parts in B-grade movies had it in him to make a big impact in films.

Brij Bhushan was an indulgent father to his only son. He did not have any opinion on the matter of Shantanu Saxena's future prospects. He allowed his son to open up the resources of BB Chopra Productions for grooming, mentoring and launching Shantanu.

His son had been uncannily right, not only in connection with Shantanu but in a few other cases during the two years or so he had directed movies for his father, before his untimely death. Shantanu Saxena's launch vehicle from BB Productions was a superhit. It made a lot of money for Brij Bhushan Chopra – and it put Shantanu on the fast track to superstardom.

The relationship between the production house and the star actor had lasted a decade, Brij Bhushan's son's death notwithstanding. Eventually, however, the inevitable clash of Himalayan sized-egos broke up this very profitable partnership.

Brij Bhushan Chopra was a round little man with enormous arrogance, a gigantic ego, and an overbearing, driving personality. When superstardom ultimately got to Shantanu's head, he could no longer digest this overpowering package with equanimity.

There was a blistering showdown during the making of what turned out to be Shantanu's last movie with BB Chopra Productions – and the actor and the movie moghul parted ways permanently, even though the film was a hit.

Now, another decade later, a vengeful and hurt Shantanu had contacted his original production house for support to resurrect his career and self-esteem.

Brij Bhushan was gratified to hear Shantanu's words. They always came back to him in this end. His stars could find their destiny nowhere else...

"Let's meet and talk about it, Shantanu," responded Brij Bhushan. "My production house is always open for you. I've just started work on a new production, a very big one, but I can consider starting another one with you."

Shantanu had screwed up a lot of courage and swallowed a lot of pride to make this phone call. He was slightly disappointed. "You've launched another picture? Then our venture could take a while to hit the floors."

"Not necessarily, Shantanu." Then a sudden blaze of inspiration hit the movie moghul. "Why don't you star in the film I've just launched? We don't have a leading man signed up yet!"

"A movie on the floors without a leading man? Is it a woman oriented subject?"

"Yes and no. The leading lady is a strong woman, all right, with a definite goal in life. But the leading actor role is quite strong. He's her benefactor in the end. We can strengthen the role further."

"Who's the leading lady?"

"Sanya Kaushik. You know her. She's acted with you."

Shantanu literally did a double take. "What? You found nobody better?"

"She's good Shantanu – very good for the role and the demands of the script. And she has an agenda. So do I. And, I think, so do you..."

They met the next day. Shantanu got a hang of the background. And realised that all three, Brij Bhushan, Sanya and he, had a similar agenda in mind – knocking Rita Sharma off her pedestal.

He had just one doubt. Would he be able to work under Dhruv Solanki again?

It turned out that he did not have to worry on this score...

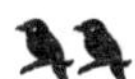

Chapter Twenty Two

BREAKING FREE

Raghu Basant's deep-set hooded eyes were half closed as he listened to his nephew. The usual cobra-like smile on his face was missing. His excellently tailored jacket did not draw attention away from his face, which was dark with anger.

"You never told me before that you were under contract with Yash Kapoor!" half snarled the dreaded mafia don.

"I had not seen the fine print, myself, when I had signed on for 'Love & Death'," lied Dhruv. "But it's there. It's a two picture binding. I'll have to do 'Story of a Superstar' for Yash, whether I like it or not. I'll direct 'Seduction' for you and Brij ji after I've completed that."

Raghu shook his head vigorously. "Can't wait till then!" His eyes were no longer half-closed. They were staring keenly at Dhruv. Raghu had the kind of cold unemotional eyes that gave a person chills. The eyes of a killer. "Break the contract with Yash Kapoor! I'll take care of the legal cases you may get slapped with. I can even arm twist that bastard Yash into releasing you."

"You will do no such thing!" Dhruv had raised his voice a notch and Raghu's eyebrows shot up. Dhruv calmed down, but only slightly. "Any intervention from your side will screw up my new found career in Bollywood. Nobody will hire a director with gangster protection! Rough arm tactics from your side on my behalf will get me black-listed by all production houses."

Raghu understood the sense of that. But he wasn't willing to lose Dhruv so easily. "Then direct both films together!" he suggested sharply.

Dhruv had anticipated this. "Can't do that. My contract with Yash specifies exclusivity!"

Raghu Basant muttered an oath. "But I had promised Sanya that you'd direct her!"

Working dangerously for his uncle for many years and being a part of the Mumbai underworld had toughened Dhruv up and filled him with an unbeatable desire to succeed. It was this toughness and inner steel that now surfaced to help him close the conversation. "Look, I gave your girlfriend a break in my directorial debut film, only on your say-so. It was a big risk, but I took it because I wanted to help her – and you. If she had turned out to be a damp squib, I would have lost credibility with my first producer, and my movie could have suffered. There's a limit to how much I can stretch myself to fulfil obligations of the past – and how much you can push me!"

There was a long tense silence. Uncle and nephew faced off each other like boxers in a ring. Anger, frustration, defiance and a sense of stalemate hung in the air like a false ceiling. They locked stares until Raghu broke it and stood up. "I don't want to break-up what we have between us, nephew," he said softly. "So, to use your words, I won't push it. Not this time. But you keep remembering how much you owe me; never forget that. You'll be directing a movie for me soon – if not my current one then, perhaps, the next. So keep yourself free for that!"

Dhruv got up and turned towards the door without comment. He wanted to get out of his uncle's lavishly appointed apartment as soon as he could. The walls of his past kept closing in on him. He would need to break free soon, or he would go mad, of that he was more than certain. But round one had gone to him; he would have to be satisfied with that for the moment..

Chapter Twenty Three
SEVERAL AGENDAS

Sanya was livid. She got the news of Dhruv's withdrawal from the project as soon as she returned to Mumbai from New York. Raghu had dropped in at her apartment shortly after her arrival to update her on the developments regarding 'Seduction'.

"Brij Bhushan Chopra has joined me as co-producer – just as Preetika had promised he would!" he first announced. "With BB Chopra productions backing us, our movie has shot into the big-league. It's now going to be a big budget extravaganza with a no-holds-barred promotional push. You're going to be a really big time star pretty soon, my love!"

Sanya's eyes had glinted dangerously. Her doll-like and incredibly pretty face had lit up with the brightness of a full moon but there was a certain amount of steel lodged behind the light brown eyes. She had every reason to rejoice at the introduction of Brij Bhushan Chopra into the equation, but the thrill at this development had less to do with her new film's prospects and more with certain other reasons that had a connection with her mother's incarceration in Rikers Island prison complex in New York City.

But her rejoicing stopped when she heard the second piece of news. "Dhruv has refused to direct me!" she exclaimed, not knowing that the actress she considered as her arch-enemy, Rita Sharma, had expressed a similar comment not very long ago in relation to her.

"He claims he's under contract to Yash Kapoor to direct one more film for him before he can consider other offers."

"Bullshit! That bitch Rita must have forced him to direct *her* picture rather than mine!"

"Well, now that you mention it, Dhruv *did* say that he will be directing Rita's 'Story of a Superstar', which is being produced by Yash..." commented Raghu thoughtfully.

There was a pregnant silence.

The silence was broken by a volcanic looking Sanya. "Rita won't get away with this!" she said in a strange voice.

Raghu's hooded eyes had turned into slits. "Can it be possible that Dhruv lied to me?" he asked, half to himself.

Sanya saw a look on her lover's face that sent a chill down her spine. "I would not be surprised," she responded viciously.

Another strained silence followed as each thought their dark thoughts. Then Sanya said: "Do you know of anybody in Yash Kapoor's office who is obliged to you and who could tell you the details of Dhruv's contract? It'll be interesting to know what the truth is – whether he is actually committed to two films for Yash as he is claiming."

"I can always find somebody who is obliged to me and who has a friend or relative in Yash Kapoor's production office," replied Raghu confidently.

Sanya got up from where she was sitting and crossed over to Raghu's sofa. She sat down next to him and put a hand on his thigh. The short man reacted immediately. He slid his arm around her, and pulled her in for a long kiss.

She let the kiss run its course, and then unlocked her lips from his. Her hand began stroking his thigh. The man squirmed slightly.

"I think you should find out as soon as you can the truth about Dhruv's contract. If he's been bullshitting you, then he must pay!"

Raghu forgot his lust for a minute. His eyes went grim. "Dhruv will learn the hard way that he cannot mess with me – if he *has* lied to me, that is!"

"Then find out fast, my love! Dhruv and Rita cannot mess with us and our film and get away scot-free. They need to get strong messages..."

Raghu momentarily ignored the hand stroking his thigh or the full lips parted invitingly and upturned towards him. "You've got a ruthless and vengeful streak in you, my girl," he observed wonderingly. "Where did you get it from?"

Chapter Twenty Four

STRONG MESSAGES

The dark brown sand of the relatively isolated Varca Beach in south Goa was soft on the feet. The sea was dark blue and the waves rolled towards the film crew in joyful abandon – one froth filled wall of water immediately followed by another, crashing on to the edge of the beach and petering out just inches away from where the lead pair of Rita Sharma and Biswajeet Kumar were enacting out a light and romantic honeymoon couple moment for the underproduction film 'Story of a Superstar'.

Dhruv Solanki ran his hand through his long hair as he sat on his director's chair a few feet away and tried to concentrate on canning perfect shots. The sun would soon be setting in the distant horizon on the edge of the Arabian Sea and time was a precious commodity – every minute to be treasured and made optimum use of. Yet, Dhruv's mind was not completely on the job at hand. He carried out his work of directing the lead actors of the film and guiding camera angles professionally yet mechanically, quite like a seasoned film director that he was fast becoming. Dhruv's mind was elsewhere. His sunglasses encased eyes hid his huge worry.

His uncle Raghu Basant had cut off all contact with him.

Whrn Dhruv had turned down Raghu's request to direct his film 'Seduction', starring Sanya Kaushik, he had expected his uncle to be angry, but temporarily. After all, he had given the don a reasonable excuse – being under a two-film contract to Yash Kapoor. But he had expected Raghu to recover from his disappointment, appoint another director, and get back to making the occasional phone call to his nephew.

But no call had been received since the day the young director had walked out of his uncle's apartment.

Dhruv, himself, had not called; in the light of his refusal to his uncle, he had not thought it to be appropriate.

But what really gnawed away at his guts was the knowledge that he had actually lied to Raghu Basant. There was no two-film binding contract with Yash. What if his uncle had found out?

The mafia don could be very vindictive and brutal if crossed. Dhruv had witnessed this on a couple of occasions in the past.

Dhruv Solanki shivered involuntarily.

"Hey, Dhruv, what's up? The shot was O.K. or not?" Biswajeet Kumar's powerful voice broke into his revere with the force of a cannon shot in a closed room.

Dhruv tried to focus on the task at hand. "Uh? Oh, yes!" He looked at the lead pair as they stood next to the edge of the sea, the waves lapping at their feet, and tried to formulate a response. The lead actors, Rita Sharma and Biswajeet Kumar, were portraying a honeymooning couple and their playfulness on the beach had been filmed using a high angle shot. For this scene, the camera had been elevated above the scene using a crane. The idea was to give a general overview, making the honeymooning couple a part of the wider scenery – the beautiful beach, the crashing waves and the slowly setting sun.

The danger of course was that, if not filmed well, the lead pair could get swallowed up by the setting in which the scene was being shot. The high angle shot could take in too much of the beauty of the scenery – and the characters could become an insignificant part of the entire shot. That would not be good.

Dhruv got to his feet. He waved to the technicians manning the levers of the crane. "Lower the crane!" he shouted. "I'll check the replay."

The crane was lowered. The cameraman, a young but talented newcomer to the film industry named Peter Salema, who was shooting his second movie, dismounted and made way for Dhruv to view the shots he had just canned on the small monitor attached to the camera – a state-of-the-art German Schumacher ARRIFLEX 235 mounted beauty.

Dhruv narrowed his mind into a single point of focus – to study the image construction of the scene that was being shot on Varca Beach. He willed all other thoughts out of his mind and studied the monitor and the images dancing on it.

It was as he had feared. He had been distracted by his problems. His attention has wavered from the task at hand. The scene had not been shot they way he had wanted it to be shot – the way it *should* have been shot.

The scene had been of a longer duration than he had wanted. The effect was of a more relaxed and slower pace while he had wanted a faster pace reflecting the sexual tension between the newly married couple. In addition, the relationship between the characters and their surroundings had become a bit skewed. The beauty of the scenery had overwhelmed the chemistry between the lead actors. This would not do...

"I'll go up now," Dhruv told Peter, smiling slightly so that the cameraman did not take his words as a sign of criticism. "Let me see if I can compose the shot a bit differently. We'll compare our output and see what works best."

Peter Salema nodded companionably and stepped away. He had understood all right, but made no comment. The film director was the captain of the ship – his word always be the final decision. If he was not happy with what had just been canned and wanted to try his hand at generating something better, then that was a call Dhruv Solanki was perfectly entitled to make.

As the crane was cranked up, Dhruv looked around at the scene below – and caught his breath. A strange man had made a sudden appearance. Even from this angle of view high up in the air, the man looked a bit familiar; in fact quite familiar. Wasn't he a henchman of his uncle?

The strange man was staring at Dhruv as the director slowly rose upwards towards the sky while seated behind the mounted film camera.

Dhruv noticed that the two crane operators on the ground were staring at this man. Then they went back to their job of operating the levers and ensuring a smooth and steady rise of the crane. The man who looked like a familiar henchman of Raghu Basant turned and walked back towards the stone steps at the edge of the beach that led to the Varca Beach Resort cottages beyond the wall of trees. It was at the Varca beach Resort that the film crew was camped for the duration of their stay in Goa.

Dhruv decided to ignore his forebodings and turned his attention to the lead pair on the ground who had, by now, freshened up with soft drinks and had put on another layer of make up as preparation for the next shot which was obviously going to be now filmed – this time by their director himself.

He waved to Rita and Biswajeet to step closer to the sea – get knee deep into the water if possible. Then Dhruv peered into the camera lens to compose the shot.

It was precisely at this moment that the crane came crashing down to the ground…

Back in Mumbai, that same day, Sunita Sharma woke from her afternoon nap with a start. Her bedside telephone was ringing frantically.

Sunita was shocked to hear her driver's frightened voice. "Madam, something terrible has happened! Can you come down to the parking area please?"

Sunita had not gone to Goa for the outdoor location shooting schedule of her daughter's new film. Her daughter had not wanted her to. A hurt Sunita had bowed to her daughter's wishes and stayed back in Mumbai, wondering sadly whether she had been right, after all, to have walked out of her husband's home in Dehradun to help her daughter pursue her destiny in Mumbai.

But now more immediate emergencies caught her full attention. Something in the driver's voice alarmed Sunita terribly. She dropped the phone, wrapped a dressing gown around her and raced out of the apartment and grabbed a lift. Once she was in the ground floor lobby area, she smelt a strange foul burning smell in the air.

Sunita hurried towards parking area. The smell got stronger – and when Sunita turned the corner she saw that the foul burning smell had been coming from a car. *Her* car. The Mercedes they had bought recently with Rita's earnings. Or what was left of it.

All the windows of the car had been smashed, the roof had been ripped off and placed on the rear seats were soggy, charred stacks of what looked like magazines. On closer inspection by the police who soon hurried to the scene, all the burnt magazines were found to be film glossies featuring Rita on their covers.

Sunita Sharma realized that day that the burned out shell of a car can be a riveting sight, even if the smoking remains are yours.

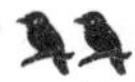

Chapter Twenty Five

PROTECTION

JP Mishra offered his protection to the beleaguered duo of Dhruv and Rita. He called up Rita the moment he read the news in the papers.

"This is terrible! Who could have done it?" he asked the young actress in a shocked voice.

Rita had been wrestling with this question herself from the moment her hysterical mother had called her up from Mumbai with the news of the damage done to their car. When she got the news she had been camping in the emergency wing of St. Xavier's Multi-specialty Hospital, the institution reputed to possess the very best medical facilities and expertise in all of Goa, waiting for Dhruv Solanki to regain consciousness.

The police in Mumbai had no clue regarding the identity of the perpetuators of this strange crime. Was it some crazed fan? Rita and her mother could think of nobody who would have any enmity with them. Why should anyone want to vandalise their car?

Then Dhruv regained consciousness in the hospital. He had suffered a hit on his head when he had fallen to the ground, along with the crane, on Goa's Varca beach, but other than that the damage was only bruises and shock.

A CT scan of the head revealed that there was nothing to worry on that front. The worry that Dhruv shared with Rita, the moment she was allowed to meet him in his hospital room, was on another front.

"I think Raghu Basant was behind the fall of the crane. I think it was sabotage!" He told her about the henchman of the mafia don he had seen on the beach during the shooting of the film.

Rita almost fainted with shock. It did not take her many seconds to put two-and-two together. "Then it must have been him behind the burning of the car, also!"

"What are you talking about?" asked Dhruv weakly, as he lay on the hospital bed, the tube of a glucose drip inserted into his arm through a needle.

When he heard the details of the burning of the Mercedes, Dhruv immediately cried: "It's Raghu all right! He's getting back at us for my pulling out of his film!"

"But why me?"

"Perhaps he thinks it was *you* who got me to dump his film."

Which was true, of course, as both knew very well.

"We'll have to ask for police protection," said Rita determinedly.

Dhruv closed his eyes for a brief moment. His torment was obvious. "No, Rita, that won't do!" he finally exclaimed weakly, opening his eyes. "I cannot reveal to the police and make public my relation and background with Raghu Basant. Yash and you now know, but this information must not go beyond both of you. If the police come into the picture, they will get to know of my past crimes. They may take action, even at this late date. And a public knowledge of all this will ruin my career! I can't risk that!"

Rita's beautiful face was pale with worry. "But the man is after us with a vengeance! Today he's hurt you and burnt my car. Tomorrow he could have us killed!"

Dhruv shook his head weakly. "No he won't. I know how he operates. These incidents were to warn us – and to pay us back for flouting his authority. I'll have to make-up with him one day, and direct his next film, perhaps. Or give some other aspiring actor a break – like I had to give Sanya Kaushik on his request."

Rita stiffened in her chair. Something began to click in her mind. "Sanya was recommended to you by Raghu Basant for 'Love & Death'," she said thoughtfully. "He's now producing a film with her as the lead actress. He seems to be quite charmed by her. The script has been written by Preetika Verma, who has no love lost for me. She's the only journalist who's thrashed my film and my acting. God knows why she hates me! Sanya doesn't like me – that was obvious right through the shooting of 'Love & Death' and during the pre-release promotional events when we went around together. Could Preetika and Sanya be trying to create competition for me? Is this film 'Seduction' and attempt to promote Sanya as my rival? Could Sanya have pushed Raghu Basant to burn my car in retaliation for your refusal to direct her and direct my film instead?"

"You mean Sanya has developed a violent hatred for you? Based on jealousy? But burning your car? She would stoop so low?"

"That would explain the burnt magazines in my vandalized car – the ones with my cover photographs!"

Dhruv closed his eyes again. "All this is getting too much for me," he said softly.

Rita was immediately concerned. "Don't think any more about all this, my love. Take rest and get back on your feet. We'll work out something..."

J P Mishra's phone call, soon after, was like a godsend. Rita was quick to grab the opportunity. She had realised, long ago, that the billionaire had a soft corner for her; now was the time to test our deeply he was enamoured of her…

"I don't know who's behind all this, J P saab," said Rita, in response to his question. "Perhaps some crazed fan. But Dhruv and I need protection. And we can't trust the police to give us sufficient cover, even if they agree to."

The industrialist, who had long been enchanted by Rita's beauty and charisma, was only too happy to offer the services of his private security agency – without any charge. "Consider the protection as part of the award you've received for your debut film," he told a far from reluctant Rita. "I absolutely insist that you accept protection from my crack team of security personnel. I am an admirer of your acting and beauty, madam," he then said unabashedly, "and feel privileged that I can extend some help in this critical phase of your career."

Rita did not know whether to be gratified by this offer and overwhelmed by this admiration. All she knew was that she was too desperate for protection for Dhruv and herself – and also her mother, in case she was also in the radar of those out to harm – and had no intention of refusing the billionaire. She agreed – and the round-the-clock security was arranged.

J P Mishra also had another reason behind his generous offer, other than a genuine desire to protect Rita, who had mesmerised him so deeply, from any harm. He wanted to keep a close watch over the director and actress couple; he wanted to know if there was anything going on between them. He would tolerate no rival for his affections…

Chapter Twenty Six

THE SOCIAL WORKER

The old man in the wheel chair had a huge scar on the right side of his shaven head – a reminder of the severe wound this road accident victim had suffered when he was admitted, near death's door, to the National Medical Institute Trauma Centre in Delhi two years ago.

Priti Mathur smiled gently at him – the old man stared back blankly.

The old man's name was Sahej Ram – at least that is what one could surmise, since these were the words tattooed on his left arm.

"Sahej Ram was in a coma for three months at the National Medical Centre," Priti Mathur informed Brij Bhushan Chopra, who was standing beside her. "He was an apparent victim of a road accident. The culprit had, of course, fled the scene," she stated matter-of-factly.

Brij Bhushan grimaced. "Where is his family?" he asked, observing a thin line of saliva beginning to trickle down from one side of Sahej Ram's mouth.

A helper employed by the old age home quickly stepped forward with a small towel and gently wiped away the saliva.

"No one knows," replied Priti. "Nobody came to the National Medical Institute Trauma Centre to claim him. Sahej Ram, himself, has never recovered from the hit-and-run accident wound to his head. He does not speak or walk – I suspect he has no memory of the past either."

As they moved away from the old man in the wheelchair, Priti pointed to a thin and shrunken old woman sitting on a stool in the garden of this special old age home for abandoned road accident victims in Mathura, located halfway between New Delhi and Agra. The old woman was mumbling away to herself.

"We call her Amma Bengali, because the attendants have overheard her muttering away in that language," said Priti Mathur. "She was also admitted to the National Medical Institute Trauma Centre with a massive head injury – she was found lying unconscious in the middle of a road, probably knocked down by a speeding vehicle. She has no known family members – it was the police who had admitted her to the hospital. She has lost her memory and does not talk to anyone. She was bedridden for a year. She can now walk around on her own – but still needs to be fed and washed."

Brij Bhushan was moved by the sight of all this human suffering, in spite of the fact that he was impatient to get on with the work that had brought him to Mathura in the first place. "Where would these poor old people have gone if you hadn't taken them in?" he asked.

"Such people have nowhere to go. That's why Jiten's father set up this special old age home in Mathura – to take in the abandoned victims of road accidents who, after treatment at Delhi's National Medical Institute Trauma Centre, are sent here by the hospital authorities. My father-in-law volunteered to look after them – and then set up this old age home."

"Your NGO has been aptly named 'Hope and Light'," commented Brij Bhushan, as Priti Mathur and he walked towards the administrative block of the old age home. "You are really doing noble work!"

"Don't let Jiten hear you – he gets very upset when people try to portray us as saints," warned Priti. "He feels that we have been gifted this opportunity to serve others; an opportunity very few get. He really feels that we are blessed to be able to do what we are doing."

Brij Bhushan said nothing. The power struggles of Bollywood, and the constant need to churn out masala entertainment for the masses that made the box office flush with cash, seemed meaningless in his present surroundings. He wondered whether he would be able to now discuss properly with Jiten Mathur the agenda that had brought him here to Mathura from Mumbai via Delhi on this sunny afternoon.

The man who the powerful entertainment moghul had come to meet was sitting behind a small desk cluttered with photographs of his late parents, his wife Priti and his two daughters. Some books gave company to the photo frames.

Jiten Mathur was forty five years of age, a couple of years older to his wife. He was dressed casually yet smartly in a light brown short kurta and black trousers – complimenting the off white salwar kameez ensemble of his wife. Jiten was mildly handsome and well built. His face had an earnest look about it – as if the man owning it felt that it would be inappropriate to enjoy life's pleasures when there was so much sorrow and suffering around. Priti had a more relaxed look on her pretty face. She seemed to posses the enviable ability to take life as it was served up and to enjoy the moment without too much concern for the unknown future.

Brij Bhushan thought that they made a very attractive couple.

Tea was served in glasses. A plate of peanuts was put on the table. The old man from Mumbai cleared his throat and began: "I've come to you to ask for help."

Jiten and Priti looked at each other. "What possible help could a person like you need?" responded Jiten, trying not to sound offensive. "And, that too, from a social worker like me?"

Brij Bhushan Chopra had left his fortress like estate outside Mumbai and made one of his rare trips to another city for the first time after two years. He had come to Mathura because the business was very urgent, one that concerned his latest film.

He needed a director. Dhruv had backed out. He needed an equally if not more talented director to replace Dhruv.

"You were one of my son's most brilliant discoveries," said Brij Bhushan.

Jiten raised his eyebrows but said nothing.

"I want you to come back to Mumbai to direct a movie for me," continued Brij Bhushan.

Jiten and Priti looked at each other again. Both carried surprised looks on their faces. Jiten turned towards the movie moghul and said: "You know I've left all that behind..."

"What a waste of great talent!" responded the old man vehemently, echoing what he and many others in the movie industry genuinely felt.

Jiten pursed his lips. His face reflected a slight annoyance. Priti hurriedly intervened. "Jiten is fully involved in running this old age home, now, Bhushan ji. He has no time to make movies."

"Why can't he hire managers to run this place? I know you can run this place on your own, Priti, with support of managers, and continue the great work. Why deprive the world of Jiten's great talent for making movies?"

"Because this is what I want to do!" shot back Jiten, unable to hold back any longer.

A brief silence followed this outburst, as Brij Bhushan steeled himself from uttering a cutting retort and burning his bridges altogether. The old and seasoned negotiator well knew when to keep his ego and arrogance in check. This was one such time. He needed Jiten Mathur; it was not the other way around.

Or was it?

Brij Bhushan Chopra had done his homework before undertaking the journey to Mathura. He knew which cards to play; he just needed to keep his patience.

Priti decided to carry the conversation forward and break the air of tension. "When my father-in-law went to the hospital for the last time five years ago, and Jiten and I rushed from Mumbai to be with him in his last hours, he expressed a wish for Jiten to carry forward his work. He didn't quite specify that Jiten should leave his career in Bollywood and run this place full time, but

Jiten felt, and I agreed, that the old age home would fold up if we didn't give it our full time attention."

"I know all that, Priti," observed Brij Bhushan, as gently as he could. "Jiten told me his reasons for leaving Mumbai and for not taking any more directorial assignments. But I had thought that it would be a temporary absence. I had thought he would settle things here and hire people to run the place and return, perhaps after a year or two. Everybody needs a sabbatical once in a while. I had thought this was his..."

Priti gazed fondly at Jiten and said: "He fell in love with the work." She waved in the direction of the window. "All those accident victims, all those old people, *need* Jiten. He is the one who is keeping them alive and that, too, with dignity."

Brij Bhushan shook his head. "No, Priti. It is *both of you* who are the saviours of all these unfortunate people. And you cannot continue doing your good work and carrying forward your father-in-law's dream under financial constraints..."

Jiten and Priti once again stared at each other. The husband gave the wife a warning look.

Brij Bhushan continued relentlessly: "I know all the details. That is why I am here. Your major funder, the Digvijay Trust, has decided to reduce the size of its grant by half, since their interest income has reduced due to the current downturn in bank interest rates. The other two foundations who have been backing you are likewise facing difficulty in continuing with their support at the same levels. The economic downturn has hit hard all trusts and foundations and CSR activities of corporates. You need fresh financial support fast, or you will have to reduce staff and stop taking in new accident survival cases."

"How-how do you know all this?" Priti looked very distressed.

"I made it my business to know all this. I wanted to know how I could induce Jiten to return to the film industry."

"You want to tempt me with money?" Jiten sounded a little hostile.

"Is that all that bad? The money will help you continue your good work, won't it?"

"Of course, it will help!" agreed Jiten, a trifle wearily. "It *is* becoming quite difficult to manage on a shoe string budget. But the flip side is the danger of my getting sucked into the film industry again – and forgetting my work here in Mathura. Film making is not a day job – it requires twenty four hours dedication and commitment and involvement of all concerned. And then one film leads to another..."

Brij Bhushan looked at his watch and decided to push for closure. "The decision is yours to make, Jiten. All I can assure you is that your fee will be on par with the top directors of the industry. I will also make a generous donation, on behalf of my family foundation – the trust set up in my son's memory – to your organisation. 'Hope and Light' will be financially stable again." He got to his feet. "Do let me know in a day or two. I will not be able to wait beyond that; I'll then approach some other director, even though you're my first choice."

It was one hour later, as Brij Bhushan Chopra was being driven back to Delhi in the limousine that had been arranged for him by his north India distributor, that the call came from Priti Mathur. Brij Bhushan felt a rush of triumph as he took the call. Yes, Priti told him, Jiten would direct the film...

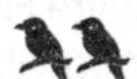

Chapter Twenty Six

RIVALRY

By the time the two under production movies had reached the half way mark in their respective schedules, the entire Hindi film industry and a large section of the entertainment media was agog with stories of the rivalry between the two projects.

'Seduction' and 'Story of a Superstar' were racing against time to get completed before each other. The two projects and all those connected with them were competing head on for the prize of public adulation and box office success.

As public interest in this rivalry grew, all other film projects underway in Bollywood ceased to matter. This was a unique happening in Indian film history; two directors were locked in battle to prove each one's supremacy over the other, two producers were competing for box office glory against each other, two lead actors were vying for the top slot in the pecking order of stardom – and two newly minted divas were out to outdo each other in blazing the silver screen with their sex appeal and unique charisma.

The last was the juiciest. Rita and Sanya had decided on a 'no holds barred' approach to proving that there could be only one screen goddess in Bollywood – and this top actress would be one of them only. To hell with the others. There was no other actress in the running now for the superstar diva crown. The biggest and best banners and teams were behind their respective movies; both were big budget projects; so only one of the two, Rita or Sanya, would capture the coveted crown – and the fight would be bitter and bloody till the very end.

Both the films were strong on story. Both films were women oriented; the stories revolved around the respective lead actresses. And each actress suited her role to perfection.

As The Girl in 'Seduction', Sanya Kaushik appeared in most of her scenes bursting at the seams in a well-chosen wardrobe that made the most of her assets, but she still managed to seem sweet and doll-like throughout. In one scene which had already been shot, she was shown dunking potato chips in champagne and thinking it was "just elegant." In another scene also already shot and quickly becoming the talk of the town with well placed media leaks, Sanya was shown keeping her underwear in the fridge to beat the summer heat.

In the past, history had been made with less masala. Now all this was super explosive.

Sanya wanted to play sex siren like it had never been played before. Her director, Jiten Mathur, who had helmed many light hearted sex romps before he had retired to Mathura, had now returned to Bollywood to find that his leading lady gifted to him by Brij Bhushan was a young woman who was skilful, discerning, cooperative, imaginative and utterly bewitching when emoting before the cameras. She radiated sex in every frame; dialogues were inconsequential. Jiten Mathur and Preetika Verma developed the script accordingly.

Rita Sharma kept tabs on the media buzz around 'Seduction' and knew she would have to stretch herself to the limit to outdo the herculean efforts Sanya and her team were making. So she stretched herself.

"I know I have this much coveted virginal and 'touch-me-not' image," the beautiful young star told her lover and director Dhruv Solanki. "But, to make 'Story of a Superstar' reach out to all audiences, if you have to make my character sit on more laps than a napkin, then please do so!"

Dhruv got the message, understood the compulsions and developed his script and storyline and characterisation accordingly.

Dhruv decided to do two things; the diva he would develop as the actress protagonist in the film would have the star appeal and charisma to reach out to the audiences from the screen, take their hand and lead them wherever she wanted them to go.

And, second, she would have love making scenes that would scorch cinema screens across the length and breadth of the country.

The first scene of the movie set the tone for what was to come. Dhruv created a poem on film, with Rita lying on her back in a bed, covered to the neck by a silken sheet. The sheet was only slightly transparent – just about enough to convey to voyeurs that, perhaps, the diva was wearing nothing else. Her thick black hair, lying loose on the pillow, was a frame for her fine features. The still shot of this scene began appearing in the initial promos and media write-ups about the film, firing up many thousands of male imaginations with the infinite possibilities in store in the film...

Regarding this opening scene, Rita would soon set the media ablaze by repeating, with a tiny change, a famous Marilyn Monroe quote: "It's not true that I did not have anything on; I had the music system on."

In tune with this brilliant start, Dhruv ensured that the sex scenes in the movie, most of them between the lead pair of Rita and Biswajeet, would get audiences blood rising and pulses racing. During one inspired schedule, he went ahead and shot one of the artsiest sex scenes ever filmed. The camera cut back and forth from intimate close-ups of Rita and Biswajeet getting very passionate in a field to shots of flowers. The extreme closeness of the camera almost made the bodies of the lead pair into abstract art, while the intercutting with the beauty of nature surrounding the lovers gave a surreal and natural blanket to what could have ended up as just another outdoor romp.

The reports of journalists visiting the sets of both films put in place very high excitement levels amongst movie buffs, of whom the country has no shortage. The stage was set for box office fireworks and major competitive activity when the movies released simultaneously on Diwali.

But the don Raghu Basant was not willing to wait for market forces to decide which of the two movies would score more...

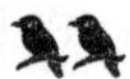

Chapter Twenty Seven

AMBUSHED

Rita and Biswajeet sat at a corner table in a plush coffee shop located on the third floor of the gigantic Ambience Mall, which is situated on the Gurgaon side of the Delhi-Gurgaon border.

Both were famous film stars with easily recognizable faces and a large fan following each. But they were not disturbed by star struck gawkers. The reason was simple: both Rita and Biswajeet were in disguise.

They were camping in Delhi with the cast and crew of their nearly completed film 'Story of a Superstar'. They had travelled to the nation's capital city for the last outdoor location of the film's shooting schedule.

Today's shooting of some action scenes in a location beyond the much hyped Delhi suburb of Gurgaon did not require the presence of either Rita or Biswajeet. So they had the day off – and the couple had decided to go shopping at Ambience Mall.

Biswajeet needed to purchase tennis shoes and clothes as well as a tennis racket and some tennis balls. He was playing a tennis star in the new film, who falls in love with the rising actress played by Rita – and he needed to do this shopping so that he could look and dress the part. The dress designer of the film would ordinarily have undertaken this assignment, but Biswajeet had volunteered to do so since he had a free day and this errand gave him an excuse to visit a mall with Rita for some quality time together. He knew Ambience Mall from previous film promotional visits. He also had relatives living in DLF City of Gurgaon, and so knew the locality well.

Rita, as was her tendency of late, had left her mother behind in Mumbai. She was gradually cutting off the apron strings that tied her to her ambitious and pushy mother, and going alone for location shooting trips was one way of asserting her independence.

"I need you to handle the business side of my affairs here in Mumbai in my absence, mother," she had told a resisting Sunita Sharma. "Let me concentrate on delivering memorable performances before the camera, for the sake of my career. Please let me not worry about the financial stuff and property matters. Please do take care of them for me – for us..."

Sunita did not have much option but to accede. Like most middle class people who suddenly come into wealth, she was suspicious of financial managers and legal advisors, most of the distrust coming from a lack of understanding of the intricacies of managing large amounts of cash. So she kept a close tab on all money transactions and understood the need to be present in Mumbai full time for this. She also had the intelligence to give her daughter, who had so quickly entered the fast track to superstardom, some degree of space which she wanted. She could lose complete hold over Rita by being too controlling, if she wasn't careful...

So Rita had travelled to Delhi without her mother. And not having any close relative or friend to keep her company, she spent most of her free time with her co-star Biswajeet Kumar.

Biswajeet had developed quite a liking for his co-star, particularly after filming certain very intimate scenes together, and even fancied that she had acquired a soft corner for him in return. He was not aware of Rita's intimacy with their director, although he had noticed their closeness and had chosen to ignore this in typical superstar single minded fashion.

Shopping over and done with, the couple had retired to this coffee shop for some much needed refreshments.

Rita *did* like Biswajeet's company. The chemistry between them was getting better and better with every passing day. Their high comfort level with each other was reflecting itself on the screen in their first film together. Biswajeet was a handsome and personable young man of about thirty two years – just ten years older than Rita. He sported long hair, a neatly trimmed moustache and an "I'm-a-stud" attitude. He joked around the sets most of the time, which Rita enjoyed very much. But he had a serious and hard working side to him, which he understated with his light hearted manner.

Rita well knew that she could get very attracted to Biwajeet, if she had a mind to. But she was in love with Dhruv – and had no reason to look for romance elsewhere.

Besides all this, her burning ambition to reach the pinnacle of success and her great desire for silver screen glory made love and relationships and commitments a secondary part of her life. Necessary, but secondary.

But the head does not always prevail over the heart.

The two young people shared similar likes and dislikes. They also shared the same profession, and understood the pulls and pressures, which they discussed in close conversations in their free time. They were both good looking and – because of their pairing in 'Story of a Superstar' – were often thrown in very close proximity to each other, sometimes in romantic and passionate enactments for the silver screen. In fact, Dhruv appeared to revel in putting the couple through extremely intimate scenes for the screen; the director had clearly taken Rita's wish to become a sex siren to heart.

The lead pair had travelled to Goa with the film crew, as well as Bangalore and Ooty. Now they were camping in Delhi. They had spent a lot of quality time together during their travels; it was a wonder they hadn't yet crossed the line...

Some of the extreme closeness between Rita and Biswajeet that their roles for their film had demanded of them just had to rub off in real life too. Theirs was a romance waiting to happen...

Today, Rita and Biswajeet shared the excitement of travelling around in disguise. The make-up artistes in the film crew had done their job well. The couple was virtually unrecognizable. Rita's jet black hair was now golden brown. Her black-and-violet pupils were covered by brown contact lenses. Her cheeks were slightly padded. She had discarded her trademark salwar kameez for a sari, in deference to her disguised state. Biswajeet now sported a goatee and thick framed spectacles which helped hide his handsome and famous face. He also wore a wig which sported a different hairstyle than his well-known and extensively copied one. The additions and changes seemed minor and innocuous – but they had transformed both Rita and Biswajeet into completely different people altogether to look at. Nobody recognized them. Nobody amongst the hundreds of people roaming around in Ambience Mall knew who they were.

Or so they thought...

For this outing, Rita had even dispensed with the security guards that had been provided to her by J P Mishra. Several incident free months had convinced her that all danger from the perpetuators of the horrific incident that had befallen Dhruv in Goa and from those who had damaged her car in Mumbai, was past. Perhaps Dhruv's fall had indeed been the result of an accident and not sabotage. Perhaps it was a crazed fan who had totalled her car – and not a jealous rival...

The mind can be convinced to believe anything.

After a relaxed session of coffee and pastries and small talk, Rita and Biswajeet decided that the time had come for them to return to their hotel in central Delhi and wait there for the rest of the cast and crew of the underproduction film to return from the day's shoot in Manesar, a small town beyond Gurgaon.

While Biswajeet paid the bill, Rita attempted to connect the number of their driver on her cell phone.

Together, they walked out of the coffee shop, shopping bags in their hands, looking like any ordinary couple – not two film stars with recent super hit movies to their credit. Out in the corridor, Rita frowned. "The driver is not picking up his phone, for some reason," she commented.

They walked towards the escalators in the centre of the third floor lobby. "Where is our driver supposed to be right now?" asked Biswajeet. "He dropped us off at the main entrance. Where did he go after that?" Biswajeet had seen Rita chatting with the driver while he was getting out of the car – so he had not bothered to involve himself in the details of how they would connect when they planned to leave the mall.

"Our car is parked in one of the basement parking areas – but the driver should be waiting for us on the ground floor, so that he can catch my phone signal on his own cell phone," replied Rita. "There will be no connectivity in the basement. He knows that. He will bring the car up to the main entrance when I call him – but I can't seem to connect."

"Keep trying – maybe our driver cannot hear his phone because of the piped music blaring through the speakers all over the mall."

Rita kept trying, with mounting irritation. She kept dialling the driver's number – but got no response.

"Shall we go down to the basement parking and look for the car?" she finally asked Biswajeet.

"How many levels of parking are there?"

"Good question!" Rita stopped in front of a security guard and found out. She turned to Biswajeet with a rueful smile. "There are three basement level parking areas!"

Her co-star scratched his head. "Then we'll have to start from the lowest level and work our way upwards. Do you know the car number?"

Rita shook her head ruefully. "No, I don't know the car number. It's a black Mercedes – there should not be that many around. We should be able to locate the car – eventually!"

Biswajeet smiled sadly. "Let's hope the search doesn't exhaust us!" He looked at the cell phone in Rita's hand. "Try to connect – one last time!"

It was no use. The driver did not take the call.

Soon, the couple was in the lower third basement. They started walking between the neatly parked rows of cars. Biswajeet held the plastic shopping bag with the tennis racket and tennis balls, shoes and clothes in his right hand. Rita held on firmly to her hand bag. She had put her phone back in the bag – it would catch no signal deep underground in the basement, anyway.

The lower third basement was unusually empty of people. Not even the parking attendants were in sight. However, the parking bays were full of cars and vans and SUVs.

It was while Rita and Biswajeet were walking slowly between a row of parked vehicles, trying to spot the black Mercedes, that it happened. There was a loud 'ping' sound as something ricocheted off the bonnet of a Maruti 800 car right next to a startled Rita.

Biswajeet stared at the hole left behind by the ricocheting object and exclaimed: "Shit!"

He grabbed the arm of a completely shocked Rita and pulled her to the ground, crouching down himself.

"What – what –?" exclaimed Rita in disbelief.

"Somebody just fired a bullet at us!" exclaimed Biswajeet, his face ashen. "We have to move from this spot right now! Follow me – and keep your head *down*!"

Rita simply could not believe what was happening. She simply followed Biswajeet in a bind daze. He was holding her arm so tightly that it hurt. Crouching low, they half ran and half walked between the rows of cars.

There was the sound of another 'ping'. Another bullet had been fired at them! And the bullet had hit one of the cars very near to them!

Rita's heart jumped to her mouth. She felt sick, suffused with dread. What was happening? This could not be for real!

She had never ever been shot at before in her life.

Bloody hell, her life was in danger!

Biswajeet dragged her along, moving faster. She began to slip as she tried to keep pace. Her sari began to unwind. "I can't keep this up!" she cried out, as softly as she could. "I can't keep on running like this!"

Biswajeet stopped. The attacker or attackers seemed to have lost them for the moment. Biswajeet looked up at the Mahindra Bolero MUV whose right side they were crouching next to. It would do…

He quickly pulled out a tennis ball from the plastic shopping bag he was holding. Rita watched in amazement as Biswajeet took out a pocketknife from somewhere inside his jacket, opened it and very quickly worked a hole in the tennis ball.

"What – what – are you *doing*?" she exclaimed breathlessly.

Biswajeet smiled tightly and said quickly: "I did a three month commando training course during my last year at college. Let's see if it pays off now!"

He reached up and held the tennis ball against the key lock of the door on the driver's side of the Mahindra Bolero, the hole in the ball facing the lock's opening.

In spite of the grave danger they appeared to be in – and her own panicked and breathless state – Rita was stunned enough to ask: "What's going on? Why have we stopped running? The attackers will catch up with us!"

In response, Biswajeet slammed his fist against the tennis ball, driving all the air out of the ball and into the key lock. Rita stared in amazement as all the four door locks popped open inside the vehicle.

Biswajeet grabbed the right side door open and pushed Rita into the Bolero. "Get to the other side, *quick*!" he instructed.

She slid over to the passenger side in an ungainly heap, her sari tearing against the gear lever and her hand bag hitting her head several times in the process.

Biswajeet was about to follow her into the vehicle when Rita's heart suddenly jumped into her mouth and she screamed: "Look out! *Behind you!"*

Biswajeet swung around. Facing him was an unshaven man with a long nose and a gun in his hand. The gun had a silencer fitted on to it – and it was pointed at the actor!

In one extremely swift movement Biswajeet pulled out the tennis racket from the shopping bag in his hand and smashed it down on the gunman's head with all the strength he could muster.

Blood spurted out from the gunman's head. He crashed to the ground.

In another swift movement, Biswajeet threw down the now broken and useless tennis racket, pulled open the rear door of the Bolero, and flung the unconscious gunman on to the floor between the seats – the blood oozing out of the wound in the head of the thug staining the rubber mats.

Rita simply stared wide-eyed at the antics of her companion, too startled to speak.

Slamming the rear door shut, Biswajeet jumped into the driver's seat of the Mahindra Bolero and poked his head under the steering column. He found the wires he needed – and the MUV's engine came to life.

A faint flutter of hope began to take birth in Rita's heart. She got some of her senses back enough to ask: "Were you a professional car thief at some point before your film career?"

Biswajeet simply grinned, put the vehicle in gear and pulled out from the parking slot.

Another 'ping' sound greeted them – this time the bullet had ricocheted off the bonnet of the Bolero they were sitting in!

A severe chill raced through Rita's body.

There was another gunman around!

Biswajeet raced the vehicle through the lower basement parking hall until he reached a bay leading upwards. He threw the Bolero into the ramp and raced up the two floors until he reached the parking ticket booth.

The barrier was down – blocking the way. The parking ticket attendant looked enquiringly at Biswajeet from inside the booth he was sitting in.

Rita prayed hard that the wounded gunman on the floor behind her would not now wake up. Why had Biswajeet pushed him into the Bolero in the first place?

Her companion pulled down the window of the vehicle and said: "I've lost the parking ticket. What's the penalty?"

Without batting an eyelid, the parking ticket attendant said: "Two hundred rupees, sir!"

Rita was quick on the uptake. She delved into her hand bag and pulled out the hundred rupee notes. Biswajeet paid up, the barrier lifted – and they drove out into the sunshine.

Rita had never before been so delighted to leave a mall.

"What now?" she asked, as they hit the highway. She looked and sounded relieved that she was still in the land of the living. But she was nevertheless tense. She turned her head and glanced nervously towards the rear of the vehicle, at the limp form lying on the floor.

"We are driving straight to the DLF City Phase-II police station – it's the nearest one, I think. Anyway, it's the nearest one that I know of! I spent a few weeks in Gurgaon last year, that's how I know. We have to hand over this unconscious gunman to the police – and inform them of the other one in Ambience Mall. The thug lying unconscious behind us will, hopefully, reveal who was behind this murder attempt – that's why I took the risk of bringing him along. Please phone somebody from the film crew and inform what happened – and ask some of our people to meet us at the DLF City Phase-II police station."

Biswajeet then looked up from his driving and grinned again. "You may like to adjust your sari before we reach the police station," he said. "Right now it's more off you than on you..."

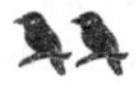

Chapter Twenty Eight

WARNING

The gunman turned out to be a hired mercenary, a killer who undertook assignments for a fat fee. He did not know the identity of the person who had paid him – in cash in small denomination notes which were kept in a suitcase hidden under a stone bench in Delhi's Lodhi Park for him to collect. He claimed he had no partner; that he had been working alone. He refused to change his stance. He had been hired over the phone. He had not recorded the number – a statement he refused to change even after severe police beatings. He was certainly a professional when it came to keeping his mouth shut in front of the police. His assignment? To finish off Rita Sharma…

In different corners of the country, people associated with Rita heard the news in shock and disbelief.

Somebody was out to kill Rita! Who could it be? And why?

Dhruv Solanaki thought he knew the answer. Yash Kapoor made an intelligent guess. Brij Bhushan Chopra had his suspicions. So did Preetika Verma. Sanya Kaushik did not need to guess – she knew.

One person decided to do something about it.

The culprit would need to be warned to stay away from Rita. And the warning would need to be effective and long lasting.

The man checked himself out carefully in front of the mirror. He had put on a wig. Now he sported very long hair, carefully slicked back with gel, and secured with a rubber band. This certainly changed his appearance considerably. He had padded his cheeks, stuck on a thick moustache over a false beard (he was probably overdoing, it but then who gave a damn?) and decorated his eyes with very dark and very large sunglasses. Even his mother would not have recognised him.

He stared at himself in the mirror for a long time, trying to look as menacing as he felt.

The eyes behind the dark glasses were passionless and blank. He violently hated the man he was going to soon meet – deeply despised him for what he had done to Rita on at least two occasions. He was cold and unemotional about what he was going to do. The person concerned had brought this event on himself – he had this warning coming to him...

Satisfied with his disguise, he swung into action.

The man rented a grey car under an assumed name. Nothing fancy. Nothing memorable. Just a plain grey Indica that allowed him complete anonymity.

He parked his car by the side of the road, in front of an empty plot of land, picked up the cricket bat from the seat next to him and got out. He locked the car and quickly strode off.

The plot of land was bounded by houses on each side. But his car was not occupying anybody's parking space, since it was standing in front of an empty plot. If anybody still had issues and raised an objection when the man returned from his errand, well that would be a problem – for that person.

It was a short walk to his destination. As the man had expected, Raghu Basant had already arrived at the spot next to the public letter box. He was impatiently looking at his watch when the man spotted him.

Raghu's cobra smile was very much in place, as was his excellent tailoring. He wore dark glasses, which hid his deep-set hooded eyes, and thick gold chains around his neck, as befitted an underworld don, a ruler of the Mumbai mafia.

It was midday. The noon sun beat down mercilessly. The road was empty of pedestrians. No cars passed by. The setting was perfect.

It was the man's phone call that had brought Raghu Basant here. The call had been made from a landline in a PCO booth. The false beard the man was wearing would ensure that the call would never be traced back to him – even if the PCO booth operator remembered his visit in the first place, which was doubtful. The identification and contact details he had entered in the PCO register were false – as was the ID proof which he had flashed to the disinterested booth operator.

The man's voice was muffled by a handkerchief when he had spoken to Raghu Basant. He had informed the mafia boss that his former mistress was in town, the one who had dumped him after he had hooked up with Sanya Kaushik. The former mistress had flown into Mumbai from Chennai that morning itself. Her husband did not know of her visit. She wanted to meet her former lover. Raghu Basant was not to try and contact her, by phone or otherwise – but simply wait for her at the spot the man had indicated over the phone. He was to come to the spot alone – no bodyguards or henchmen, please. She would drive up and pick up Raghu for their rendezvous.

The man was her new secretary, he had informed the surprisingly gullible don. She had asked her secretary to fix the meeting.

Raghu Basant was still besotted with his former southern film star mistress – the reigning queen of the Tamil movie industry. He drank up the man's story like a thirsty person in a burning desert who has been offered a bottle of chilled beer.

Love is not blind as much as lust is. Lust blinds all the senses and deadens the brain.

The fool had walked so easily into the man's trap…

The man stroked his false beard one last time. It was firmly in place. He walked over to where Raghu Basant was standing, next to the red painted public letter box.

"Hello!" said the man cheerfully.

The mafia don had been looking the other way, trying to spot his mistress and her car. He swung around with a jerk, his face a complicated mixture of confusion, irritation and slight nervousness. "Did you speak to me?" he asked.

"Yes," replied the man.

Raghu Basant did not respond. He waited for the strange man to make the next move. The expression on his face was now a mixture of puzzlement and caution. He stole a surreptitious look at his watch.

"I want to talk to you about Rita Sharma," the man continued.

The don's jaw dropped. *"What!"*

"Yes, about Rita. Why are you trying to harm her?"

Even though he was wearing dark glasses, the man could sense Raghu Basant's eyes flashing with anger. "Who – who *are* you? What do you want?"

"Stop trying to harm Rita. Lay off her!"

Raghu's face went purple with rage. "Are – are you *mad?* Who the hell *are* you?"

"You've asked that question for the second time. Who I am is not important. What's important is that you will make no further attempts to hurt, injure or kill Rita Sharma. *Get it?*"

The gangster drew a deep breath. "Look mister – I don't know who you are or what your game is, but if you don't get lost from here, I'll call the police!"

"I don't think you'll do that. What if your mistress turns up while the police are talking to you? What if the cops recognise you for the underworld don that you are – and decide that the opportunity is ripe to take you to the police station for some conversation regarding your illegal activities?"

Raghu Basant went white. His jaw dropped again. "H-how – what – how…" was all he managed to stammer out.

The man decided to insert some firmness into the proceedings. "Look, let's stop wasting time. My request to you is a simple one. Stop trying to harm Rita. Can't you promise that much?"

The don struggled to find words. The man's heart sank – he could make out that Raghu Basant would not cooperate so easily. The man felt sad.

"You're-you're *mad* – and I'm getting out of here!" Raghu almost shouted.

The man sighed. "So you won't listen to me?"

Raghu's puffed up face was contorted with rage. *"Get lost, you asshole!"*

The man did what had to be done. He raised the cricket bat and then brought it down with great force and smashed it hard into Raghu Basant's right kneecap.

The mafia king collapsed to the ground with a blistering scream of pain. Fortunately there was no one on this empty side street to witness this drama. The don lay there on the pavement writhing in agony, thick beads of sweat quickly gathering on his forehead, his face grimaced with the severity of the pain from his broken knee. His sunglasses had fallen off – and there was fear in his eyes. Naked fear.

The man knelt down besides the fallen underworld don. "No more attacks on Rita Sharma or on anybody else or on anything around her," he told Raghu Basant quietly but firmly. He spoke in low measured tones and with controlled menace. "Otherwise, I will hunt you down and smash your other kneecap also."

The king of the Mumbai underworld said nothing. He simply stared at his attacker with horror stricken eyes.

"And yes, another thing," the man continued. "If you report this to the police or send you goons and henchmen after me, your romance with your former mistress will become public property. Your current mistress Sanya Kaushik will get to know that you tried to meet her today – and so will your former girlfriend's husband."

The man then got to his feet and gave the parting shot. He pulled out the photograph from his jacket pocket. "You have a lovely girlfriend. She has a beautiful, doll-like face. Don't force me to disfigure it. Her movie career will finish instantly, and you'll have to search for a new heroine for your film, even while I find you and break your other leg, or worse…"

The man turned and walked off, the photograph back in his pocket and the cricket bat held firmly in his hand. He hoped his negotiating technique would not fail…

It was now time to deal with the woman.

It was a couple of hours later. Sanya had rushed out of the fancy restaurant in which she had had been having lunch. An agitated phone call from a henchman of Raghu Basant had alerted her that her lover was in hospital. The details were not clear, just that he had been attacked by somebody. Could she come over? He was conscious and asking for her...

An acquaintance strolled out of the restaurant, while Sanya was standing on the pavement, waiting for her car to arrive, and waved at the actress. Sanya waved back absentmindedly, then turned around to see if her car had arrived. Her bodyguard, supplied by Raghu, stood a couple of paces behind her.

Suddenly, a Scorpio SUV raced by, and somebody sitting in the passenger seat leaned out of the window and flung the contents of a can of paint at her! It hit Sanya straight on, almost knocking her to the ground.

The jeep shot away, and Sanya could hear somebody screaming with laughter.

As her bodyguard rushed up to her, his face a mask of shock and horror, people quickly gathered around Sanya and stared at her in amazement, as she stood there dripping red paint...

Chapter Twenty Nine

COUNTER MEASURES AND A TRUCE OF SORTS

Brij Bhushan Chopra was almost choking with rage as he spoke. The words shot out of his mouth like bullets. His eyes blazed.

"This-this is most certainly not the kind of publicity I need for my film!" He waved agitatedly at the pile of newspapers stacked untidily in the middle of his gigantic desk.

Preetika Verma and Sanya Kaushik squirmed in their seats. Shantanu Saxena looked dazed.

"The newspapers are full of stories about the murderous attack on Rita and Biwajeet in that mall in Delhi! Everybody is speculating about who hired that gunman who was captured! The damage to Rita's car and the injuries Dhruv suffered in Goa are now being linked to some overall conspiracy theory. Now we have that paint attack on Sanya – there is speculation that this also is linked, like some kind of retaliation move. That means that fingers are being pointed in our direction for the troubles befalling those associated with 'Story of a Superstar'! My film has become entangled in some kind of gangster warfare situation – and I will not tolerate this!"

All eyes turned to Sanya. The reference to 'gangster' was clearly directed at her boyfriend and the co-producer of 'Seduction'.

Sanya's pretty face was ashen. It had finally dawned on her that actions also provoke reactions. The paint attack on her was shattering. What was more devastating was the information from Raghu; the man who had smashed his kneecap so brutally had done so in clear retaliation for the earlier attacks on Rita and the others!

Whoever he was, Raghu's attacker knew the source of the earlier attacks; it was no secret as Sanya had foolishly believed.

What was all the more horrible was the fact that Sanya had only known of the crane incident in Goa and, of course, the car arson attack in Mumbai. *She had not known of Raghu's plans to kill Rita and Biwajeet in Delhi!*

Sanya had a horrible vision of her great dreams of stardom ending up in a prison cell...

Sanya also now realised that ruthless attacks worked both ways. That Rita's camp could also hurt and brutalise was a shocking revelation. *Did Rita herself order yesterday's attacks on Sanya and Raghu?*

Sanya realised that the other three in the room were staring at her. She pulled herself together and said: "Raghu will be out of action for a long time. He's in hospital. He's promised me that he will not take retaliatory action..."

Preetika looked startled. "Why's Raghu in hospital?"

Sanya told them.

Brij Bhushan's face turned apoplectic. The old man appeared to be on the verge of having a fit. Preetika turned pale and Shantanu's eyes bulged in disbelief.

"Are you serious?" roared Brij Bhushan. "Somebody from Rita's camp has bashed up Raghu because he tried to kill her? Is this some kind of an insane joke?"

"Raghu's kneecap is shattered, all right. He didn't do it himself!" responded Sanya sharply.

The tense silence that followed was thick enough to cut with a knife.

Then Brij Bhushan got to his feet slowly and pointed his finger menacingly at Sanya. The short round old man looked like a powerful volcano on the point of eruption. "I have put in ten crore rupees into 'Seduction' already. I will not lose this money because you and your gangster boyfriend decided to bring underworld strong arm tactics into film business and failed." He drew a deep breath, collected his thoughts and proceeded. "Do you realise that all of us in this room could become implicated in Raghu's mad attack on Rita and Biwajeet? Do you realise that the destruction of Rita's car could land up on your doorstep, and rightly so? What if the police investigations to the crane accident in Goa lead to Raghu? Who will pay for all the consequences? *It is I and my investment that will take the hardest hit! My reputation will be in shambles. My money will go down the drain! I will not allow that to happen!"*

For a wild moment Sanya thought that the movie moghul was about to pick up something from his desk and throw it at her. That moment passed. But the old man was not finished.

"You will inform Raghu that he is no longer associated with 'Seduction'. He is no longer the co-producer of this movie. I will pay him back all his investments and terminate my agreement with him."

Preetika and Shantanu looked expectantly at Sanya, who nodded her head slowly. The old man was right – this was the correct thing to do in the light of the circumstances. She did not know how she would convince Raghu, but she would do it. Her career was more important to her than anything else. Nothing would come in the way of her career, not even Raghu.

"Brij ji is right," commented Preetika, a trifle unnecessarily. "We need to distance the movie from Raghu Basant, and from all underworld connections."

"I'll see to it!" responded Sanya shortly.

"I'm not finished." Brij Bhushan turned his finger towards Shantanu. "You and Sanya will begin an affair together!" he commanded.

Shantanu's mouth fell open. *"What?"*

Sanya stared at the old man, then at the actor and then back at the movie moghul. "What are you *saying,* Brij ji?"

For the first time that afternoon, Brij Bhushan Chopra smiled. It was a grim smile, but a smile nevertheless. He looked like a gross thick penguin who had been hit by a pleasant thought.

"You don't find Shantanu attractive?" he asked, his eyes narrowing.

Of course Sanya did! Who wouldn't? But manufactured love?

It was as if the old man had read her mind. "I'm not asking you to jump into bed with Shantanu, my dear, though I don't know what's holding you back." Sanya looked as if she was about to protest at this gross statement, so Brij Bhushan raised his hands in a placating gesture. "Hear me out, before you say anything! All I'm asking you two to do is to *behave* as if you're having an affair and give the media opportunity to speculate that some of your on screen chemistry has spilled over into real life. If not the real thing, at least you can *pretend* to be love birds while the movie is under production, and a little beyond! This will help the film's prospects, take away attention from the present stories of attempted murder and mayhem and de-link Sanya from Raghu."

"You're – you're simply brilliant, Brij ji!" exclaimed Preetika, jumping to her feet in excitement. "This off screen romance will focus public attention squarely back on our film – and keep it there. I will fill up my columns with stories of this sizzling romance! Sanya and Shantanu's love story will become the talk of the nation. This will turn around our fortunes..."

"And Raghu will hopefully fade into the background..." observed Brij Bhushan. "That is essential! His continued connection with our film and with Sanya will spell disaster!"

Shantanu stole a glance at Sanya out of the corner of his eyes. He had always appreciated her beauty, of course, and had greatly enjoyed all the romantic scenes they had filmed together so far. Enveloping her in a couple of kisses for the screen had been extremely pleasurable. Her full lips were very kissable and she had engaged in the lip lock scenes with full vigour, opening her mouth wide and actually allowing him to invade it with his tongue, for a passionate effect on close-up shots. But his mind had always been occupied with thoughts of Rita, his heart obsessed by her memory, his body burning in desire for her, while his brain at the same time plotted her downfall. This had not allowed him to look beyond – at the possibilities inherent in his current co-star. But now...

The movie moghul was still not finished. “Good!” he exclaimed. “That's settled then. And now, I have a task of my own...”

The other three looked enquiringly at him. What now?

“I will pay a visit to Yash Kapoor's office,” continued Brij Bhushan unexpectedly. “It's time I built some bridges. The world needs to see that I have no enmity with the makers of ‘Story of a Superstar’...”

Chapter Thirty

PSYCHO

The man watched Brij Bhushan Chopra leave the office building of Yash Kapoor with mixed feelings.

The white haired movie moghul had a relieved look on his face as he entered his chauffeur driven limousine. A tenuous truce – actually, an understanding to contain extremist elements in each other's camps – had been arrived at. The shooting of the remaining portions of both the underproduction movies 'Story of a Superstar' and 'Seduction' would now proceed uninterrupted, or so it was hoped.

The man well knew the other reason why the movie moghul had met the producer of Rita's film – to try and douse all rumors that Brij Bhushan himself was behind attempts to destabilize Yash's movie project. But the man was not so easily fooled. Everybody connected with 'Seduction' was an enemy of Rita. Recent events had confirmed that beyond any doubt. Rita was lucky to be alive after that murder attempt!

The man promised himself that she would not face such danger again. *Never!* He would see to that!

The man remembered the way he had smashed the kneecap of that thug Raghu Basant. He shivered with pleasure at the memory of the sharp crack he had heard when the cricket bat he had wielded had connected with bone. A wave of excitement coursed through his veins as he recalled the look of naked fear in the eyes of that powerful king of the underworld as he lay there on the road, powerless, helpless, in pain…

The man needed release. The activity of the previous day with first Raghu Basant and then that bitch Sanya Kaushik had left him filled with nervous energy. He had to expend it. He thrilled at the memory of the manner in which he had chucked the paint on Sanya! Her look of shock was to be seen to be believed! He had found the whole episode immensely funny; to be repeated again at an opportune moment.

But now, the release…

He needed release urgently. And there was only one way for this – the only way he knew…

He knew which bar in which hotel to go to. He had picked up whores from there before. He was always heavily disguised on such outings, of course, and this added to the sense of power. He knew who they were but they did not know who he was. Wouldn't they be surprised if they did?

"I like your style," she said. "I can sleep with you this afternoon, if that's what you want – but it'll cost you!"

She was in her thirties, with short dyed brown hair and a suntanned face which probably indicated a fondness for the swimming pool or the beach. She had on a blue t-shirt with a deep cut neck downwards, very short denim skirt and white ankle boots. From what he could see, her body was good and she was pretty in a cheap way.

The man's hands began to itch slightly. "How much will it cost me?" he asked.

She looked the man over carefully. They always did. Their greed and stupidity were both unbelievable, thought the man. This one was being quite obvious. She would love to fleece him – but she didn't want to quote a price which would shock him and make him discard her. The man decided to put her out of her misery.

"Ten thousand bucks for the whole afternoon and night. If you have another appointment for the night, then drop it!"

The woman tried to look nonchalant, but the sudden excited gleam in her eyes gave her away. She shifted her mini skirted bottom slightly on the bar stool and uncrossed and then crossed her bare legs again, in a crude attempt to indicate to the man the numerous pleasures that he would be earning in return for his generosity. She leaned forward slightly so that he couldn't miss her impressive trademark cleavage.

It was her neck that would bring the man pleasure – not her legs or any other part of her anatomy. But the stupid woman would learn this only when it was too late for her to do anything about it…

The man took out a bundle of five hundred rupee notes held together with a rubber band – he never carried a wallet when out on a 'job' – and counted out and handed her six of them. "Here's an advance," he said. "Just a token – to assure you that I'm serious." Then he gave her the details of the nondescript hotel and the room number she would need to go to in an hour's time, separately – and not together with him.

As he stepped out of the bar a little later and began walking down the street towards the car he had rented for the afternoon and the evening, the lines of the song travelled through his mind: *"And another one bites the dust…"*

The love making was not bad, actually. The woman was quite a pro. When he leaned down and kissed her full on the lips, her body started to come alive. She pulled him to her and locked him in a tight embrace as her body sought to match his rhythm. They climbed the peaks of ecstasy together and climaxed simultaneously.

The man actually felt a little sorry when he reached out for the soft and smooth neck moments after the passion had subsided and she lay trembling under him. As the trembling from the love making subsided, a terror began to grip her as the horror of what was about to happen dawned on her. The fear in the eyes was the same as in the two earlier cases. The scream was killed before it could burst forth. The man enjoyed strangling her – that evil peddler of flesh, destroyer of goodness, wreaker of lives. As the woman weakened and the struggling against the inevitable end slowly ceased, his mind compressed itself into a single lightning bolt of hatred. As he throttled out another life, he screamed out in a combination of ecstasy and terror: *"I shall avenge, avenge, avenge! Help me – dear God, help me!"*

Chapter Thirty One

PAIRING

Rita Sharma returned to the film sets shaken and mortified but also filled with a stronger resolve to overcome all obstacles that came her way and complete the movie she well knew would cement her rule over the Hindi film industry.

She was now surrounded by round-the-clock security, most of it provided by her billionaire admirer J P Mishra but there was also a police commando always by her side.

Having so narrowly escaped death, Rita had now re-discovered her love for her mother. Sunita Sharma was once again Rita's constant companion on and off the sets – except when she was closeted with her co-star Biswajeet.

Their stunning experience in the basement parking of Ambience Mall in Gurgaon, and Biwajeet's equally astonishing presence of mind during the crisis, had brought the co-stars very close to each other. Rita had fallen in love.

Being held in Biswajeet's arms every day on the sets, being kissed by him, being fired up by his ambition, charm, talent and immense sexuality, Rita had become smitten.

But she was also into a passionate relationship with her film's director who she had hero-worshipped since her first movie with him.

Rita was at a crossroads in her personal life, and she would need to resolve her dilemmas quickly. But she did not let her professional life get effected by her emotional turmoil. She put her heart and soul into her portrayal of a superstar in the making, a role which had such close echoes with her real life...

On another set in another studio, Sanya too focused all her attentions on the lead actress role she was playing in the sex comedy romp that was touted to make her the new sex symbol of Bollywood. If there was a distraction, it was her well orchestrated and very public display of affection for her co-star Shantanu, a lot of it actually stemming from a growing closeness in real life to this handsome, charming and troubled superstar.

BB Chopra Productions put the full force of its clout with the media to develop public interest in the love affair of the lead pair of its new movie. Brij Bhushan's PR department went into overdrive. Carefully posed photographs of the couple were distributed widely. The publicists worked hard on their contacts and arranged for joint TV interviews of Sanya and Shantanu as part of the promotional activity for the film 'Seduction' which was rapidly nearing completion, in a neck-and-neck race with Rita's 'Story of a Superster'. Press interviews regarding the film project, wherever possible, were given together by the star couple.

And then Brij Bhushan had a brainwave. A new movie from the BB Productions stable was due for release. It was called 'Om Shanti' and starred a couple of newcomers. The movie had been very long in the making due to the illness of its lead actress, but was now ready for release. Shantanu had a very small walk-in part, a 'guest appearance' in film business parlance. He had been brought into the project, for a reasonably big fee completely disproportionate to his minuscule role, in order to add the much needed star quotient to a project otherwise low on star power. Shantanu had shot for the movie a year ago – and had completely forgotten about it. Brij Bhushan decided to use the premiere of the film to officially launch Sanya and Shantanu as a couple in love.

Sanya was to be Shantanu's date for the premiere of 'Om Shanti' at the Raj Kamal theatre in Bandra.

The decision to pair them off at the premiere for the benefit of the media cameras was made by Brij Bhushan and orchestrated by the publicists of BB Chopra Productions, but given their growing fondness for each other Shantanu and Sanya were happy to oblige.

Everyone knew that Shantanu hated these occasions, but paired with Sanya and with her company throughout the event, he might be able to get through the experience, it was felt. Shantanu knew the importance of going to the premiere with Sanya; it would greatly help their movie 'Seduction' if the film glossies depicted them as a real-life couple and it would firmly take away all attention from her earlier association with the don Raghu Basant.

They arrived together at the venue of the premiere in the same long black limousine. Stepping out on to the red carpet, they set off an immediate explosion of camera flashbulbs and cheers from the crowd. Inside the theatre, as Shantanu squirmed in his seat, critical of his performance, Sanya told him he was nuts. She thought he was magnificent during the few minutes he actually appeared on the screen. When it was over, he grabbed her hand and rushed out of the theatre and into the waiting limousine before the crowds could get to them...

At the post-premiere party at a glitzy restaurant in a popular five-star hotel, the star couple drew everyone's gaze like a pair of magnets. "The combination of their beauty was staggering," gushed a famous film journalist in a newspaper feature the next morning. In fact, that day and for many days in a row, the page three sections of most newspapers and practically all film glossies were filled with breathless reports of their love affair.

Brij Bhushan Chopra, the producer of 'Seduction', the publicists and marketing experts in BB Chopra Productions, and the director Jiten Mathur, were all thrilled at the publicity, hoping to ride it through to the film's release. The large number of stories in the press also bolstered the efforts to turn Sanya into a full-fledged star in the same league as Rita Sharma.

It wasn't long before Preetika Verma also got into the act, striding onto the sets one day, wearing her usual designer baggy pants and loose fitting jacket, her hair perfectly coiffed and groomed to within an inch of her life. She had come to watch the day's shooting, in her capacity as the movie's story and scriptwriter, and peered from behind the camera as Jiten shot Shantanu and Sanya in a romantic clinch. "Sanya did the old Madhubala trick," she told her readers the next day in her columns. "She took him. She mesmerised Shantanu completely. Not a carpenter, electrician, prop man or labourer left the set. Some even sat on ladders to get a better look. That girl Sanya gets them all – from 15 to 50. What a dish!"

Chapter Thirty Two

MADE FOR EACH OTHER

What happened next was, perhaps, inevitable.

As the film neared completion, Shantanu and Sanya became inseparable. Then, one day, Sanya decided to take the bull by the horns. "I know you do drugs," she told Shantanu.

They were sitting in Shantanu's well appointed make-up van, chilling out after a hard day's work. The star smiled grimly. "You know and so does the rest of the world. So? Why are you bringing it up? You dislike those who dope?"

Sanya reached out and gripped his hand. She squeezed and said: "I do drugs too."

Shantanu was immediately interested. "You do? Wow! Who would have guessed?" He looked questioningly at her and she nodded her head slightly. Words didn't have to be spoken; they understood each other quite well now...

That evening, when Shantanu Saxena went back to his mansion on Carter Road, he had company. Sanya Kaushik was with him, and she had made all arrangements for their highly anticipated evening of drugs and drinks.

Sanya Kaushik, soon to be crowned a queen of Bollywood, not only knew how to enjoy getting stoned – but she also knew all the best and most reliable drug suppliers in town.

She had learnt a lot as mistress and lover of Mumbai's underworld king Raghu Basant, and she was going to put her knowledge and experience to good use that evening.

One of the prominent drug suppliers of Mumbai was now sitting with Shantanu and Sanya at one corner of the massive dining table in the Carter Road mansion. His name was George. He had been carrying a Gucci satchel when he had entered the Carter Road mansion, which he now placed on the table. He had 'professionalism' written all over his face – no small talk, no being in awe in the presence of a superstar, no looking around in appreciation of the lavish surroundings. Just business.

"How many eight-balls do you want?" he asked Sanya, who had summoned him a little earlier with a phone call.

Sanya looked at Shantanu, who made a face. "Just make sure that we don't run out of supply!" the superstar responded.

Sanya did a quick mental calculation. "Five eight-balls should do it," she finally said.

George stroked his goatee and then opened the Gucci satchel. He rummaged inside and eventually produced five small plastic containers which he then carefully placed on the dining table – in front of the couple. "Here are your five eight-balls."

Both Sanya and Shantanu understood what the slang 'eight-balls' meant. Each of the five plastic containers contained an eighth of an ounce, or three-and-a-half grams each, of cocaine.

The market value of the contents of the five small containers was about eight lakh rupees.

Sanya reached out to pick up a container – but George stopped her with a steely look through his thick framed spectacles. "Money first, please!" The 'please' was added in deference to the presence of the superstar – otherwise George was known to be quite caustic with his vocabulary.

Almost by magic, the star's safari suited secretary materialized. He carried a thick wad of bank notes in his hand. "Come with me," he said.

George was assured by the sight of the wad of bank notes in Vivek Budhiraja's hand. He pushed back his chair, got up, picked up his Gucci satchel and turned to follow the secretary out of the room. "Have a great party!" was his parting comment.

Shantanu just grunted. As Sanya reached out for the cocaine, he pulled out a pipe from his shirt pocket and placed it on the table. Sanya picked it up and opened a container. The fine white powder shined in the glow of the room lights. This was pure cocaine – not street cocaine, which was cut with other substance to increase profits for the drug dealers.

She filled the pipe with the cocaine powder and lit it up. Shantanu took the pipe from Sanya – and then proceeded to get wasted out of his mind…

At eight in the evening, the drinks and drugs party which had begun around the dining table in the ground floor dining room later shifted to the mini-theatre located on the second floor of Shantanu's Carter Road mansion.

In the mini-theatre, a third dimension was added to this cosy party for two; x-rated films.

The couple then spent several blissful hours smoking cocaine, drinking scotch whisky and watching blue films. They eventually hit the master bedroom.

They stood by the door and began kissing, their bodies pressed closely up against each other, the heat rising. The kisses they exchanged were hot and slow, fast and exciting. Kissing hadn't been this much fun for both of them in a long while.

Their pent up desire for each other then exploded. They were soon on the bed, their clothes strewn all over the floor. Their passion set fire to the bed. When he kissed her, she opened her mouth wide and he invaded it with his tongue. She drew him down to her with a fierceness that was part passion part desperate need. "Shantanu, Shantanu," she whispered, her voice gaining in intensity, until she rose up beneath him in one last climax of passion. When it was over, she lay trembling in his arms as Shantanu kept repeating in a whisper: "Where the f**k have you been all my life?"

Chapter Thirty Three

A DESPERATE MAN

The double-storied shack called Lucia's Hell is located on north Goa's Anjuna beach. It is a flourishing restaurant-bar-hookah joint that is popular with Goa's large and growing expatriate population for several reasons, the foremost being that people openly peddle and consume drugs inside – activities legally banned in Goa. The local police are paid off handsomely by the politically well connected owners and so they turn a blind eye. The shack Lucia's Hell is home to regular rave parties – and loud music is played in its hashish filled atmosphere till very late into the night, all days of the week.

Tonight was no different.

The second floor bar area was dimly lit. The overall colour of the lighting was a dark shade of red. It gave the interiors an eerie and ghostly kind of feel and look that matched the steady thump of trance music pulsating through the heavy duty speakers.

There were foreigners everywhere. Hippies with dreadlocks and backpackers lounged about on plastic chairs or sat sprawled on the floor. Many were taking drags from opium sticks – which were being passed around like toffees in a children's birthday party. The smoke-filled air was laden with intoxicating smells. The crush of bodies and the beat of the rhythmic music added to a mesmerizing ambience.

A middle aged and dishevelled man of clearly Indian nationality sat hunched up on a plastic chair in a corner of the second floor bar and restaurant of Lucia's Hell shack and tried to make conversation with the African drug peddler John between low points in the loud music.

"A gram of cocaine will cost you two thousand eight hundred rupees, my friend," said John as he blew smoke rings in the air. "Ten grams of ganja will cost you one thousand rupees. I can also give you an Ecstasy tablet for six hundred rupees."

The unkempt and untidy looking Indian man John was speaking to began to look desperate. He was Shakti Singh, former senior actor of the Indian film industry. He was completely unrecognizable from the days he had adorned the silver screen as anti-hero in some films and outright baddie in others – it is doubtful whether any of his former fans would recognize him as he was now.

His thick and very long black matted locks had not been washed for days. His beard was also thick and long and very unkempt. Thick lens spectacles covered his eyes. He had worn no beard or spectacles when he had starred in and swaggered through umpteen B-grade movies till just about three years ago.

This was before he had tried to rape that young and pretty aspirant for Hindi film stardom, Sanya Kaushik, in the hotel he had owned in Mumbai.

Shakti Singh had clearly fallen on bad days. The hooked nose was still in place, but the eyes were no longer that of a predator. The eyes, rather, carried a kind of hunted look, like those of one who had lately been at the receiving end of many punches by an unkind fate. The kurta pyjama ensemble he sported had not been favoured with a wash for many days; the sandals on the feet were a bit tattered.

Shakti swallowed hard, assumed a pleading air, and was about to respond to the African drug peddler when, suddenly, a bare-chested, heavily tattooed foreign man of seemingly north European origin sitting at the other end of the large room screamed in a drug-induced haze. The foreigner's mahogany face was frozen like a waxwork, or a facelift gone wrong.

Nobody looked in the direction of the screaming foreigner. What was happening was quite common here. Shakti had his own problems – he couldn't give a damn.

The foreigner lapsed into a sullen silence. The music again took over the senses with its overpowering force and rhythmic thumping. The beat was certainly hypnotic, Shakti thought to himself, momentarily forgetting his desperate need. Then he turned his attention back to the African drug peddler.

John wore the glazed look of a hard core heroin addict. His arms were pincushions of needle jabs. Shakti had come to the shack looking for 'doctor' John – the African's regular use of hypodermic syringes had earned him the nickname 'doctor'. John epitomized the drug trade in Goa. He was both consumer and retailer. Proceeds from the sales he made also helped fund his own daily fix. Drugs were also often traded by him for sexual favours – particularly from the many Russian women who landed in Goa in droves during the winter tourist season, looking to make a fast buck, if not serious money.

Shakti had run out of his small store of drugs. He needed to stock up immediately. And he needed a fix urgently – withdrawal symptoms were already setting in. There was a danger that soon he would be screaming violently and tearing at his hair and rolling on the ground if John did not oblige him. Would he?

Shakti began stuttering. He was scared as hell that the drug peddler would turn him down. "Can – can you loan me a fix, my friend. I – I don't have cash on me right now. I – I'll pay you later, tomorrow perhaps?"

John froze. His lips grimaced into what looked like a snarl. "Not happening, bro. I deal in cash, not credit!" He struggled to his feet.

Shakti desperately grabbed his arm. "Don't go, *please!* I – I need a fix badly..."

The pupils of John's eyes turned into red spots. "You think I'm running some kind of charity outfit, *asshole*?" He shook off Shakti's hands and growled. "Stop bugging me! You know the rules of the game – cash for dope..."

Shakti jumped to his feet. He was swaying slightly. "I don't have any cash left. The guy who was sending me money from Mumbai has stopped taking my calls. Give me something to do, *anything*, and I'll do it for you. Just give me some dope, man, just a little bit!"

John's glazed eyes ran over the defeated man in front of him. He began to look a bit interested. *"Anything?"* he asked speculatively.

Shakti was perspiring now, very tense and very anxious. *"Anything – just anything!* Tell – tell me what you want me to do!"

"You'll go to jail for me?"

"Uh?"

"Jail, man jail! My inside man in Arthur Road jail in Mumbai has just come out. My trade with the prisoners has stopped. You'll go in? You'll be my inside man?"

Shakti eyed the man warily. "Will I get dope inside the jail?"

"All you want, man. For yourself – and for sale. You'll make a lot of money, man – you'll be rich when you come out..."

"What – what do I have to do to go in?"

John laughed. "Rob a bank, man. Rape a woman. Kill somebody. It's not very difficult!"

Shakti thought that one over. As the music blaring all around him pulsated with its steady beat, Sanya's face once again flashed before his eyes. There was not a day during the last three years when he had not thought bitterly of her.

She was the bitch who had slapped him when he had tried to rape her. She was the bitch who had then taken that photo of him on her phone camera, as he had lunged at her bare-chested, with knife in hand. The photo which that bastard Ragu Basant, to whom he was already deeply in debt, had later used to blackmail him into signing off the hotel to him for peanuts, and who had then driven him out of Mumbai with threats of getting him arrested for attempted rape and murder using that very same photo as evidence.

It had been all downhill for him since then – while that bitch and that bastard had prospered...

It had been difficult to miss all those film magazine covers displayed on the racks of the newspaper vendors in the markets and beaches of Goa. Sanya Kaushik was featured regularly; she had clearly attained her goal of film stardom pretty fast. She was often seen smiling at the world from those covers, and posing provocatively in skimpy dresses. Yet that bitch had gone all coy and upset and violent with him when all he had wanted was a little fun with her in return for a role in one of his films...

She would pay!

They would all pay; Sanya, Raghu – and even that bastard Vinod, his secretary, who had taken on the responsibility of selling off Shakti's few assets like cars and shares and sending the proceeds to Goa to help him survive in his anonymity. Vinod had stopped sending money for a long time now – and was not even taking his calls. That traitor! That fraud! He would pay for his treachery!

But first Shakti needed to survive. He needed to eat. He needed a way to pay for his daily drug fixes, without which he would soon be dead. Where would he get the money for all this?

John had offered him a way out of his desperate situation. Yes, he would go to jail – work for John while inside jail. He would make money from selling drugs to his fellow prisoners. His needs would also be provided for this way; he would get money and drugs...

And to get into jail, he would commit a crime. He would take his revenge on that bitch Sanya – who was responsible for having ruined his life. A revenge that would last, a revenge whose consequences would make her wish that she had never been born.

She may have forgotten his existence by now, but he would remind her of him. The time had come. After all, as Shakti remembered from one of his once popular dialogues, wasn't revenge a dish best enjoyed when cold?

Chapter Thirty Four

PRE-RELEASE PROMOTIONAL ACTIVITY

The school buses started dropping off the children on Marine Drive, the three kilometre long boulevard in south Mumbai that fronts the coastline with the Arabian Sea and connects Nariman Point with Malabar Hills, from around eight o'clock in the morning. At this relatively early hour, scores of people were taking a refreshing saunter on the esplanade and enjoying the magical sight of the sparkling waters of this natural bay of the Arabian Sea. The cool breeze from the ocean caressed with its gentle touch. The branches of the palm trees lining the road swayed slightly in the gentle morning breeze.

It was a picturesque start to the last leg of the promotional events preceding the Diwali day release of the much hyped movie 'Story of a Superstar'.

The managers and executives of the PR company that was in charge of promoting the film were out in full strength. They had been overseeing the arrangements and logistics for a couple of hours already. The producer of the film, Yash Kapoor, was also present in Marine Drive with his team, having driven down from his north Mumbai residence a little while ago.

Since the buses could not park alongside the pavement of the boulevard, arrangements were made for the school children arriving earlier to sit in groups and enjoy refreshments like soft drinks and snacks. It would take a while for all participants of the charity walkathon from all the fifteen participating schools to arrive and gather at this starting point on Marine Drive opposite the Air India office tower. Some of the buses were coming to the venue from as far away as Thane on one side of the megapolis and Navi Mumbai on the other side. It would take an hour or so for the gathering to be complete.

T-shirts, some with "Children are Superstars" written on them and some with "Put all children in schools" emblazoned on them, were distributed amongst the arriving school kids, who changed into them in specially built enclosures on the side of the pavement. Prior permission for this gathering and for the march by children had, of course, been taken from the traffic police and municipal authorities well over a fortnight ago. The application letter had mentioned that the event would be "a walkathon for charity".

The media contingents had already arrived at the Marine Drive starting point in full force. This was expected. Advance press notes had specified that the walkathon would be graced not only by the stars of the soon to be released film 'Story of a Superstar' but also by the reigning king of the Indian film industry, Aamir Khan. Today would be another exciting day for the addicts of star studded events.

TV trucks lined the road – with their huge dishes facing upward into the clear blue sky. Journalists and reporters of all shapes and sizes and ages mingled amongst the assembled children, taking sound bites and making notes for the stories and features they would eventually file on this event.

The police were there, of course, but more in the capacity of protectors of the children from any untoward happening, rather than law enforcers or crowd controllers. There was no question of any rough and dirty activity against school children, certainly not in such a public gathering and in the midst of this entire media glare.

The traffic police were out in full force. They had been informed of the route. The march of the school children would culminate – where else? – at the park in front of the one hundred year old Regent theatre where Rita Sharma's new movie would premiere. The traffic police would regulate traffic on the entire five kilometre route. If any child got injured by a vehicle on the road, the media would come down on the traffic police like a ton of bricks. No, the Mumbai traffic police would definitely not risk such an eventuality.

The event was being organised to further the cause of 'Educate A Child Foundation'. Each school contingent was being backed by a corporate house with a CSR budget to spend. The funds would go to the NGO's programme which arranged sponsorship for street children to attend school and also livelihood opportunities for their parents, to prevent them forcing their children to drop out and become street vendors or beggars again.

No film release in Bollywood history had ever been associated with such a cause or event. It was a simple yet brilliant concept – a win-win situation for all. The film stars brought in the media, and gained from the media attention in turn. The publicity hungry corporate houses and brands shelled out sponsorship to the school contingents for the cause in return for the guaranteed publicity the event would garner. All event banners and stage backdrops carried the logos of the sponsoring corporate houses and their brands. The school children would walk for a cause, gather points for social service, earn t-shirts, feed on sponsored snacks and have a good time with their friends. They would also appear on TV.

The NGO managers would get a windfall of funds for their programme – and publicity for their cause.

And 'Story of Superstar' would get unique pre-release publicity and the benefit of association with a social cause. The stars associated with the event would get a leg-up in image building with their public.

Placards with catchy slogans extolling the cause of child education and written in clear bold lettering by 'Educate A Child Foundation' activists were distributed among the school children in large numbers.

At nine in the morning, almost to the minute and as per schedule, the film star Aamir Khan, that great champion of social causes, arrived along with Rita Sharma and Biswajeet Kumar and Dhruv Solanki in a cavalcade of cars. He jumped out of his limousine wearing dark glasses, jeans and a t-shirt. His bodyguards immediately surrounded him in a tight circle. Rita, Biswajeet and Dhruv were close behind, bodyguards in tow.

Rita was her usual radiant self, and all male eyes in the vicinity fixated on her. The cameras captured her scintillating smile and sparkling eyes and reporters strained to catch her attention for quick sound bytes. But the security minders present in large numbers kept them at bay. There would be a press conference at the end of the walkathon, in the Regent cinema theatre premises; all opportunities for media questions would then be made available.

The children gave a roar of approval and almost broke ranks. Their focus of attention was Aamir and, to a lesser extent, Biswajeet. The teachers and 'Educate A Child Foundation' staff and PR agency employees stretched themselves to the limit to keep the children in the orderly lines that they had been arranged into for the march.

Yash looked pleadingly at Aamir. "Could you quickly walk down the lines of children and shake as many hands as possible? That's the only way they'll stay in their lines…"

Aamir Khan grinned broadly. "Of course! Let's see if you can keep pace with me!"

Aamir did not walk down the lines of children. He *ran* down the lines of children. The speed with which he shook hands with the delighted kids was phenomenal. Yash and Biswajeet were huffing and puffing a bit within five minutes but the guest superstar for the event looked as fresh and fit as when he had started. Rita and Dhruv had wisely refrained from joining the male superstars and their producer in their handshaking marathon with the children.

Job done, the three men quickly ran back to the front of the long line of school children, standing four to a row, in their bright t-shirts. They joined Rita and Dhruv. There were about nine hundred children gathered there that morning to participate in the charity walkathon – about sixty kids per school. PR agency executives handed Aamir Khan, Rita, Biswajeet, Dhruv and Yash the flags with which they would kick off the march. The largest was reserved for Aamir, the chief guest of the event, who was present in his capacity as Social Ambassador of the NGO 'Educate A Child Foundation'

Aamir Khan raised the flag, which had "Children are Superstars" painted on both sides, high in the air – and then brought it down with a flourish.

Many dozens of camera flash bulbs popped. The television cameras focused on the superstars, focused on the children, focused on the t-shirts and placards and on the messages they carried and swept the entire dramatic tableau with the sparkling waters of the Arabian Sea in the background, into hundreds and thousands of TV sets across the country. The images would be re-telecast throughout the day and well into the night.

The great march of school children to raise funds for the education of thousands of children from poverty stricken backgrounds had been flagged off.

This promotional event for the movie "Story of a Superstar' was a grand success well before the walkathon ended...

Chapter Thirty Five

REVENGE

The warm afternoon sun of what had been a pleasant Mumbai autumn day added to the glow that lit up Shakti Singh's brain and heart.

Shakti's hair was no longer unkempt. The drug dealer John had financed a shampoo wash and a haircut – and other improvements. The beard was now neatly trimmed; the clothes were new and clean. The spectacles were firmly in place, the face was impassive.

Shakti Singh did not stand out in the crowd. He merged in well. He was just another faceless fan, waiting for the stars to arrive.

His body, however, throbbed to enter a great battle. His whole being was elated that his deed would be seen by several hundred thousand TV viewers all over the country.

In the elastic waistband of his tennis slacks was a small pistol, concealed by the zippered jacket pulled down to his crotch. That white jacket blazed with vertical red lightning bolts. A blue-dotted scarlet bandana bound his hair.

In his right hand he held a huge, silvery Evian bottle, though it contained something other than spring water. Shakti Singh presented himself perfectly to the showbiz world he had left three years ago and which he was about to now re-enter in great style.

That world was a huge crowd in front of the Royal Cinema House in downtown Mumbai, a crowd eagerly awaiting the arrival of the film stars of the newly released and about to be premiered and much anticipated movie 'Seduction'. And also awaiting the arrival of the superstar guests to the event.

Specially erected grandstands held the spectators; the street itself was filled with TV cameras and reporters who would send iconic images all over India. Tonight people would see many of their favourite movie stars in the flesh, shed of their manufactured mythic skins, subject to the emotional high and real-life euphoria of a film release.

Uniformed security guards with shiny brown batons tucked neatly in holsters formed a perimeter to keep the spectators in check.

But Shakti did not worry about them. In his heydays, he had been an action star, used to enacting many screen stunts on his own. Despite his downhill slide of the last three years, he was still bigger, faster and tougher than those men, and he held the great and unbeatable element of surprise. The people he was wary of were the TV reporters and camera persons, who fearlessly staked out territory to intercept the celebrities. But today they would be more eager to record than prevent. Or so he hoped.

A white limousine pulled up to the entrance of the cinema theatre, and Shakti saw Sanya Kaushik "the sexiest woman in Bollywood," as many film magazines were already calling her. As she emerged, the crowd pressed against the barriers shouting her name. Cameras surrounded her and transported her beauty and sexual grace to the far corners of the country, small towns and big. She waved.

Shakti vaulted over the grandstand fence. He zigzagged through the traffic barriers, saw the blue shirts of the security guards start to converge, the pattern familiar. They didn't have the right angle. With surprise still on his side, he slipped past them as easily as an expert footballer evading his tacklers. And he arrived exactly at the right second.

There was Sanya talking into a reporter's microphone, head tilted to show her best side to the cameras. *The bitch! What a pro she had become at the film star game!* Three bodyguards were standing beside her. Shakti made sure that the cameras had him in their frames, and then he threw the liquid from the bottle into Sanya's face.

He shouted: "Here's some acid, you bitch!" Then he looked directly into a couple of TV cameras that were now focussed squarely on him, his face composed, serious, and dignified. "She deserved it," he said. He was immediately covered by a wave of blue-shirted security men with their batons at the ready. He knelt on the ground.

At the last moment, Sanya Kaushik had seen his face. She heard his shout and turned her face and instinctively bent her head.

The liquid flew over her head and some of it hit the left cheek and ear of the bodyguard who had been standing right behind her.

He screamed out in pain and shock. The acid quickly burnt off the skin where it landed. Fortunately for the bodyguard, most the acid missed him. All of it missed Sanya.

Hundreds and thousands of people saw it all on TV – and would continue to see it in replay after replay on their television screens for many days and weeks to come. The lovely face of Sanya Kaushik, encased in shock and horror – and terrible recognition when she saw her attacker; the look of true fear that followed – the bodyguard's scream of pain.

The same hundreds of thousands of viewers watched as the police dragged Shakti off. He looked like a movie star himself, as he raised his shackled hands in a victory salute, only to collapse as an enraged policeman, finding the gun in his waistband, gave him a short, terrible blow to the kidney.

Sanya Kaushik, still reeling from shock, shouted for help for her fallen bodyguard, whose face had gone all red, whose eyes were puffed up. People were crashing all around her, to protect her, to carry her away.

Help arrived in the form of a few standby medics from the emergency medical team camping in a police ambulance in anticipation of possible accidents amongst the teaming crowds. The bodyguard was quickly carried away for urgent burns treatment. But the injuries were minor, the medics were able to assure the reporters and a relieved Sanya.

Sanya Kaushik, showing great courage, then walked into the theatre as if nothing much had happened. She smiled and waved to the crowds as she did so – and won a million fans.

She looked strong and cheerful, unmindful of the recent attack and the terrible consequences if the acid had found its mark, but deep in her heart she was terrified.

As for her film – it was now pre-destined to be a super hit.

Chapter Thirty Six

JEALOUSY

For the Indian film industry, it was a unique Diwali weekend, followed by a unique week and a unique month. There were two super hits, running neck-to-neck in the race for audience eyeballs – and neither cut into the other's business, as had been feared when the plans for a simultaneous Diwali release had first been announced. Moviegoers and movie going families saw *both* films. *Both* movies garnered record breaking initials ('Seduction' a notch higher than 'Story of a Superstar') followed by record breaking first week collections ('Story of a Superstar' a tiny bit ahead of 'Seduction'). By the end of the first month, it was clear that *both* films would eventually enter the much coveted and elite hundred crore rupee club, a double first for women oriented movies.

Two new screen goddesses had been crowned in Bollywood, who had both managed to, in a short period of time, far outstrip – in fan following, market price, box office standing and critical acclaim – all other actresses of the immediate past and the very present.

They had started out together in the same film. Then, with their second and separate films, they had managed to carve out famous and unique identities for themselves for both their on screen and off screen personas.

Rita Sharma was once again hailed as the quintessential beauty who possessed a grace that took everybody's breath away; an incandescent beauty who, according to a famous film critic, "just shone and shone and shone..."

And Sanya Kaushik? Across the land there was, for her, according to an article in 'Star, Style and Sizzle' magazine, a loud and sustained wolf whistle emanating from the doors of the nation's garages and gyms, college hostels and bachelor pads. That wolf whistle, accompanied by howls of outrage in certain quarters, became positively deafening when her links with the infamous underworld don of Mumbai Raghu Basant and her closeness to Bollywood's 'bad boy' Shantanu Saxena became well known due to the investigative efforts of some intrepid journalists.

This is when big problems started for Sanya. Really big problems.

Raghu Basant was furious as hell. "What the f**k is all this about – these stories about you and Shantanu?" he shouted over the phone, after reading a titillating story in a film glossy.

Sanya gripped her telephone instrument so tightly that her knuckles gleamed. "All bull shit!" she lied, quaking inwardly. "This sort of gossip comes with the territory, Raghu, you know that. Stars are soft targets for yellow journalists."

"There's no smoke without a fire!" retorted Raghu unoriginally. "There's too much talk of this. You haven't bedded him, have you?"

There was a pause. "Of course not, Raghu! Don't be ridiculous. He was my co-star and so we got close. You're aware of that. We kissed many times for the screen; you were OK with that. It never got personal." Sanya quickly changed the subject. "What are you going to do about that madman Shakti Singh? He almost destroyed me with his acid attack! Are you going to let him get away with it?"

Raghu Basant did not reply in a long while. That pause before Sanya's answer had told him everything. A cold rage gripped him, but he controlled himself. He would need to play smart to regain what was rightfully his; Sanya was now a big star who would need careful handling. But, first, he needed to attend to Shakti; Sanya was absolutely right about that…

Chapter Thirty Seven

CONFRONTATION

When one side in a relationship acquires fame and iconic status, equations are bound to change. It is resistance to this change from the other side which can assume frightening proportions.

In the world that revolved around Rita Sharma, it was the freshly minted diva herself who pushed the 'change' button in all her relationships.

When Rita promptly followed up her phenomenal success with her second movie by signing up another film with Biswajeet Kumar as her co-star again, several people saw red.

Her mother was one of them. "You never consulted me!" she accused during a showdown over dinner one night.

Rita was cool. "No mother, I did not consult you. And I don't see the need to consult you before taking such decisions."

Sunita swallowed hard. Her face reddened. "How *dare* you talk to me like that, Rita! Are you forgetting that it is *I* who brought you to Mumbai and into films? Are you forgetting so quickly all the hard work and long hours I put in to further your career, all the humiliations I faced, all the networking and bulldozing I had to do?"

Rita threw down her napkin and got angrily to her feet. "Don't be ridiculous mother! You pushed me into films to fulfill *your* dreams as well as mine. Well, now that your daughter's a big star, learn to bask in the glory. Yes, you surely deserve to. But our equation has changed now, mother. I'm the star and I'm the one who will take all decisions regarding my career. You're welcome to stay on here in Mumbai and in my house as my support and, of course, as my mother. But I don't need you as my manager – I've hired a professional to fill that job. I also don't need you as a secretary – I have a seasoned one. My finances are being managed by expert advisors. So, mother, thank you for all your support so far, but that's it! Let's stay friends and on good terms. Else, it's your problem, not mine. Dad's house in Dehradun may be a happier place for you than my home in Mumbai..."

As Sunita's mouth fell open and a sudden rush of tears welled up in her eyes, Rita strode out of the dining room, meal unfinished.

Dhruv Solanki was more difficult to handle. "How – how could you go and sign a new movie without first checking with me if I had a project ready for you?" he asked Rita over a phone call he hurriedly made the moment he heard the news, his agitated voice crackling over the long distance connection. He had gone to Ahmedabad for a few days to celebrate his second straight directorial success with his immediate family. His mother had long ago forgiven her prodigal son for having run away from home to go to Mumbai to seek his destiny, and she now happily celebrated his massive success and rising wealth.

Rita tried to be patient. "It's a *professional* decision that I have taken, Dhruv, in the interest of my career. I feel that Biswajeet and I make a very good onscreen pair, and I liked the story which Brij ji narrated to me. More importantly, I want to make up to Brij ji. He got back at me for not working with him and signed on Sanya. Look at what wonders this has done for her career. I don't want him to get fixated on her; I want him to consider me an equally important asset for his production house."

"So now you're working for BB Chopra Productions? *The enemy camp?*"

"There are no enemies in the film world, Dhruv. I could not work with Brij ji earlier because I was under a two-film contract with Yash. The two films are over, so now I can. I like the project; I need to build an association with BB Chopra Productions; I don't want Sanya to monopolise them; so I've signed up."

"Just like that? You have quite a calculating and shrewd mind, don't you?"

"I've been told that before."

A pause.

"Why am I not directing it?"

"Brij ji has decided on Dheeraj Chauhan."

"You did not push for me?"

"It was Brij ji's decision to take, not mine. Besides, I think he signed on Dheeraj Chauhan before he approached me."

"But – but I left the 'Seduction' project of Brij ji on your say so! I walked out on Brij ji and my uncle to direct you in 'Story of a Superstar'! How can you now ditch me and join Brij ji's project?"

"You *wanted* to direct 'Story of a Superstar' – that's why you rebelled against your uncle's diktat, Dhruv," retorted Rita, not choosing to remember how she had seduced the besotted director to dump his project with Sanya Kaushik in favour of hers.

A selective memory is often an ambitious star's best friend.

Dhruv was beside himself with shock, anger and resentment. "How can you be so calm and collected about this, Rita? I directed your film because I love you. I have risked my uncle's enmity, Brij ji's anger, Sanya's resentment only on your behalf – for you and on your say-so! Now, you're singing a different tune! Have – have things changed between us?"

Rita could not answer this. Her near death experience in the basement parking of Ambience Mall in Gurgaon, and Biwajeet's equally astonishing presence of mind during the crisis, had brought the co-stars very close to each other. Yes, Rita had fallen in love with Biswajeet, in spite of already being in an intimate relationship with Dhruv.

Being held in the young and handsome Biswajeet's arms every day on the sets of 'Story of a Superstar', being kissed by him during their romantic scenes together, being fired up by his ambition, charm, talent and immense sexuality, Rita had become smitten. She had not slept with him yet, but she knew that it was only a matter of time before even that happened.

The truth was that she had signed on for the new movie 'Love Struck' not just because she had liked the story and had wanted to work with the production house of Brij Bhushan and was attracted by the remuneration, but also because Biswajeet was in it and he had asked her to team up with him. How could she have refused?

The silence dragged on and Dhruv lost patience. "I'm coming back to Mumbai tonight, Rita. I need to talk to you face-to-face about this!" He abruptly cut the connection.

Rita turned to Yash for support – only to end up in another confrontation scene.

"You're going to work for Brij Bhushan Chopra? You're deserting *me*?"

Rita could not understand it. Everybody seemed to think they *owned* her.

"I'm deserting nobody, Yash. I had a two-film contract with you. That's over. Now I'm free to sign up with whoever I want. Why is this so difficult for everybody to understand?"

"Brij is my competitor!"

"Not mine."

There was a very tense silence. For the first time since she had known him, Rita saw Yash really furious. He looked ready to explode – violently. She decided to quickly end the conversation before things got out of hand. They had met over coffee in the exclusive roof top club of the Citadal Hotel overlooking the Arabian Sea. "I'm leaving, now, Yash. I have a script reading session with Dheeraj and Biswajeet. I'll be late, if I don't go now…"

Yash Kapoor did not have the time to react. She was gone.

Rita did not know it, but she had set in motion a series of events which would re-shape the face of the Mumbai film industry.

Chapter Thirty Eight
RETRIBUTION

Jealousy drives you nuts. Makes you do crazy things. Jealousy makes you lose all reason. Jealousy is all encompassing.

Rita had driven two men to jealously, insane jealousy, the kind that burns everybody and everything it touches.

Sanya had also aroused a similar passion – in the breast of a very dangerous man.

Raghu Basant was now driven by this madness. He knew, *just knew*, that Sanya was cheating on him. Not only he – the whole world seemed to know of the affair between Shantanu and her. Somebody would *pay...*

But, first, that revenge seeking rogue Shakti Singh would pay – for daring to dream of avenging himself against Sanya and, perhaps later, against Raghu.

It was not long after Raghu had made up his mind that jail guards at Mumbai's Arthur Road prison discovered Shakti after a long search. He had been missing from the roll call taken in the evening after the prisoners had returned to their barracks from the evening physicals in the courtyard. The alarms had rung and the security systems had swung into action. Even a cat would not have been able to leave the Arthur Road jail complex without detection.

Not that Shakti had any plans of leaving the jail. He could not, even if he had wanted to. When he was discovered lying in a remote corner of the prison complex, he was very dead. He had apparently been kicked to death by several strong legs wearing heavy boots. Practically every bone in his body was broken. Though it was never conclusively proved, it appeared that several of the prisoners in the jail, who were never identified, had, for some reason, ganged up against Shakti and beaten him to death...

It was with grim satisfaction that Raghu telephoned Sanya and gave her the news. She did not know whether to be happy – or terribly frightened.

Her former lover's immense clout had once again been manifested. He could, it seemed, bribe anybody he chose, wherever and whenever he wanted and get anything done. This could be bad news for Shantanu and her...

Shantanu had to be warned. And quickly.

The superstar was camping in New York. He had gone there for an advertisement shoot. His stock was high after his latest success and he was much in demand for ad films and movie projects. The films would take time – Sanya and he wanted to act together and so they were scouting for appropriate scripts. But ad films were a lucrative immediate option; they also kept stars in the public eye till their next movie.

Sanya was scheduled to join Shantanu in New York at the fag end of his filming schedule, and also use the opportunity provided by that trip to see her mother. Her visa was ready. She now preponed her trip to New York.

Shantanu was surprised but pleased with her unexpectedly early visit. He met Sanya at the airport and enveloped her in a warm embrace. Their drive to the hotel in the rented chauffeur driven limousine was made in comfortable silence, interspersed with passionate kisses. Sanya had no intention of spoiling the first few hours of meeting between the lovers with unpleasant talk of her former lover and her incarcerated mother. There would be enough time for all that...

Once in the hotel, they lost no time. They started kissing as soon as they entered their suite, leaving Sanya's bags ignored and unattended. They soon found themselves in bed, enveloped in each other's arms. Their love making was without the violent urgency of those meeting after a long gap. They were gentle with each other, letting the climax build slowly until they reached the crest, then, together, in one joyous bonding, they surged down the long lane of light, swiftly and silently, blotting the world out in their moment of glorious ecstasy.

When it was over, they lay very close together, hand-in-hand, as their bodies slowly ceased to tremble and as a sense of deep calmness and peace settled in. She snuggled closer to him – and began speaking.

Shantanu digested everything with quiet calmness, very maturely and soberly. Love had changed him a lot. His first thoughts were for the mother. "Why is she in jail?"

"For murder."

Shantanu digested this in silence. Then: "Who did she kill?"

"My mother does not speak much, never about this. The prison records are sketchy – she killed some Indian man here in New York."

"How old were you when she was jailed?"

"A baby."

Shantanu turned on his side and looked at her. "Who brought you up? You grew up in jail?"

She grimaced. "Thankfully, no. My mother's younger sister lives in Bangalore; she and her husband brought me up. They have no children of their own."

"And you met your mother, for the first time after you grew up, just a year ago?"

"Yes, after my debut movie – and after signing on my first film as leading lady. My aunt had told me of my mother's starry aspirations in her youth and her attempts to break into Bollywood. She was not as lucky as me; so I wanted to meet her after getting the success she never got in films. I wanted her to see her dreams fulfilled through me."

"How – how was your first meeting? How did it go?"

Sanya was silent. Then, after a few beats, she said: "Come with me to Rikers Island tomorrow, Shantanu, and see for yourself how she is..."

They were both silent for a little while more. Then Sanya raised herself up and stared into Shantanu's eyes. "There is a reason, Shantanu, why I got better breaks than my mother in Bollywood. I had a godfather."

He raised his eyebrows. "You just told me about him – Raghu Basant. Why are you telling me this again?"

"It concerns you – us. We are in grave danger!" Then she told him about Raghu's anger on learning about their affair.

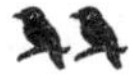

Chapter Thirty Nine
COMPLICATIONS

It was J P Mishra who saved Rita from Dhruv.

At first he was furious to learn that there had been a relationship between the director and the diva. Rita had turned to the billionaire industrialist in desperation, having found Yash to be as opposed to her tie-up with BB Chopra Productions as Dhruv. Reluctant to involve Biswajeet in what was turning out to be a messy tangle between her and her present associates, she called up the tycoon for support, knowing his fondness for her. After all, he was already picking up the tab for her personal security.

J P Mishra dropped everything and landed up at Rita Sharma's plush apartment.

"I will explain to Dhruv to face facts," he assured her gravely, "but have you considered that, perhaps, you should also reconsider your actions, the manner in which you relate to people around you?"

Rita looked startled. "What do you mean, JP?"

He pondered over his reply and then said in measured tones: "Can't you see that you were and are and will continue to be, an irresistible man magnet? You draw men to you, talented men, brainy men, passionate men – and they fall head over heels in love with you. The consequences can be quite devastating when these men realise that they are not the centre of your universe..."

Rita was not prepared for this kind of a sermon, but realised the validity of what had been said. "It's difficult to keep a check on such emotions, JP," she responded seriously, "particularly in the world we film folk inhabit. We are constantly thrown in the company of beautiful and talented people, we worked in close proximity with them, enact romantic scenes, discuss passion as routinely if it were a piece of stationary. Emotions do tend to get tangled up in such circumstances; it's not new for the film industry!"

JP Mishra nodded at this. He was not finished however; he had his own agenda to pursue. However, further discussion was stalled by the arrival of an extremely agitated looking Dhruv Solanki.

The director looked meaningfully at the tycoon and then at Rita. "We need to talk," he told her, his face flushed. "In *private.*"

JP Mishra got to his feet and said quietly. "You'll do all your talking here, young man, in my presence."

Dhruv flushed a deeper red. His eyes burned holes into Rita. "What – what is the *meaning* of this? Who is *he* to interfere between us?"

"He's a close friend, Dhruv. Don't forget that the bodyguards surrounding you and me have been provided by JP. I'm not comfortable around you any longer. He's here to support me against any unreasonable behaviour on your part."

For a tense minute it looked like Dhruv might take a swing at the tycoon. Then he thought the better of it. He pointed a finger at Rita.

"I know you're dumping me, Rita. But you won't get away with it so easily. Success seems to have gone to your head. You can't use and abuse people like this! You will work only in my films and for nobody else! You cannot link up with anybody else while I'm around!" He stared hard at JP Mishra. "I know you and your kind, mister. If you're fishing in troubled waters, it's because you have your own agenda with Rita. Well, you'll not get what you want. She's mine forever!"

Before either Rita or JP Mishra could react to this startling volley of words, Dhruv turned on his heels and stormed out of the apartment, almost colliding with Yash Kapoor, who was entering through the open doorway.

Dhruv ignored Yash completely and rushed out, face red and eyes blazing.

Yash stared after him and then looked inquiringly at Rita and JP Mishra. "What just happened?" he asked.

Rita told him.

Chapter Forty
THE MOTHER

Sanya and Shantanu stepped into a small room and waited for the grim looking guards to open a sliding door. There was an uncomfortable silence as the guards executed this simple act. As the door slid open, the couple stepped into a large hall.

There were about twenty five or so round tables placed in the hall. Each table had three chairs assigned to it. The young woman knew from the experience of earlier visits to the Rikers Island jail complex that one of the chairs was meant for the prison inmate and the other two were for the prisoner's visitors.

Most of the tables were already occupied by inmates chatting or sitting in silence with relatives or friends.

Most of the inmates in this visitors hall of the prison complex of New York City were either white or black American – or of Latin American descent.

There was only one Indian in the room – the young woman's mother.

Her mother was seated at a table in one corner of the hall. Her face was hidden in the shadows – a grim reminder of the deep darkness that had engulfed the middle aged woman's life.

Sanya bit her lips as she spotted her mother. She gave a quick look at Shantanu. The handsome film star was looking very grim. This was a touch of real life he had never experienced before. Sanya forced herself to push down the anger that had suddenly begun welling up inside her against the merciless fates and events that had brought her mother to this unholy place – to be incarcerated like a dangerous and wild animal, for her whole life.

Her mother did not look up as she approached his table. She had not done so during the past two visits.

The guards kept a watchful eye on the threesome as the young woman and the tall man reached the table, pulled a chair towards the older woman and slowly sat down. Sanya forced out a bright smile. "How are you, mother?" she asked the older woman.

Radhika Kaushik kept looking down at her hands, which were placed formally on her lap. She had shrunk further into her clothes since Sanya had last seen her. Her closely cropped hair, cut as per prison regulations, gave her face and head almost a skull like appearance – like Nazi concentration camp prisoners looked in feature films and documentaries. The young woman shivered involuntarily.

Shantanu looked a bit dazed, and very uncomfortable.

The woman they had come to see was perhaps only a couple or so years older to him in years but physically the age gap was about a dozen years or more. Sanya's mother was in her mid-forties but looked ten years older at least. Shantanu, like a true film star, had maintained his appearance to look several years younger than he actually was.

Sanya looked at her mother and shivered again. She could not help it.

This momentary shiver brought a spark of life in Sanya's mother. Slowly she raised her head and looked blankly at the daughter who had come to America, all the way from India, for the sole purpose of visiting her mother in jail.

Sanya was carrying in her hand several film glossies. These had been carefully screened by the prison guards before they had allowed Sanya to carry them into the jail complex and then into the visitors' room. The fact that Sanya's photograph featured in all the covers of the film magazines she was carrying had convinced the guards that there was no covert reason by the visitors for carrying them into the prison.

Sanya placed the film magazines on the table between herself and her mother. "I'm a star now, mother," she said softly. "A big star of the Hindi film industry."

Radhika Kaushik stared at the magazines. She slowly reached out and picked up the top one. She gazed at the photograph of Sanya on the cover. The girl looked beautiful and seductive, and very glamorous. Radhika placed her right hand on the picture and carefully caressed it. Then she said softly: "And to think your father did not want you to be born."

At first Sanya did not think she had heard right. "What did you say, mother?" she asked, not believing her ears.

Shantanu had also heard Radhika. This strange woman in front of him was beginning to look a bit familiar, but for the life of him he couldn't imagine where he could have seen her before. "Your daughter has made you very proud. She's the queen of Bollywood, now."

Radhika lowered her head. Her shoulders began shaking. Sanya looked stricken. "Mother, please don't cry. Aren't you happy for me?"

Radhika's shoulders continued to shake. She sobbed quietly. Shantanu and Sanya looked helplessly at each other and let the sobbing continue.

Finally, the sobbing subsided. When Radhika raised her face again, it was transformed. There was a light in her eyes which had not been there before. She looked younger, stronger. Shantanu stared hard and marvelled; there was a distinct similarity in looks between Radhika and Sanya, in spite of the devastation that years in prison had wrought on the older woman's face.

Again the thought struck him. Where had he seen Sanya's mother before?

"I am glad I have lived to see this day, my child," she said softly. "Destiny has been unkind to me, but whatever has happened has happened for the good. God has been kind to you, girl; don't misuse your good fortune."

Sanya's eyes bored into that of her mother. "What did you just say about my father? Who was he? Aunt never told me; she said she did not know."

Radhika took time to reply. Her eyes went blank; her mind had flown back to some memories of the past. Then she spoke, in a clear and firm voice. "Your aunt does not know. Only two people know. Me, of course, and a close friend of your father's who thinks my child was born dead.

"Where is my father?"

"He's dead."

Shantanu put a protective arm around Sanya, who slowly asked with a shaking voice: "Who was he, mother? When did he die? How did he die? Please tell me..."

Radhika closed her eyes. She began to rock in her chair.

Sanya leaned forward. A sudden lightning rod of illumination had flashed in her mind. Tears of anger, deep grief and desperation welled up in her eyes. "This man you killed, the man whose name the prison records show is Devendra – was he my father?"

When he heard the name, Shantanu's eyes widened with astonishment and shock. Now he remembered when he had met Sanya's mother. That knowledge shook him to his core.

After a devastatingly painful silence, the older woman nodded her head slowly. "Yes, I killed your father..."

Chapter Forty One

TWO DECADES AGO

When Radhika opened her eyes, she immediately realized three things. One, she was not alone. Two, she was not in her own bed. Three, she had no clothes on. It was then that she recalled the previous night.

She turned to her right. Yes, he was lying next to her on the bed, in deep sleep.

Her head throbbed. Spying her clothes on a chair, she crept quietly out of bed and gathered up her things. She spied a door that could lead to a bathroom. She scurried over to it and turned the knob. Yes, she was right. She quickly entered the bathroom and shut the door quietly behind her.

Once dressed, she felt more secure. She splashed water on her eyes, dried her face with a towel and re-entered the bedroom.

He was awake and sitting up on the bed bare-chested, the sheet pulled modestly up to his waist. He saw her and grinned. "Good morning, sweetheart!"

She stared at him. She remembered his sweet words of the night before at the studio party, how well they had danced together, how high they had got on dope and alcohol and then landing up here, in this hotel room.

"Good morning." She decided to wait for him to make the next move, to indicate to her where they would go from here. Had it been just a one night stand for him, this hot shot film director and great hope of Bollywood?

He saw her hesitate and patted the bed with his right hand. "I see you're dressed and ready to go somewhere. What's the hurry? Come and sit here, sweetheart. Let's talk of us..."

Radhika was encouraged by this. But he kept referring to her as 'sweetheart'. Did he even remember her name?

He did. When she sat down by the edge of the bed, he reached out and stroked her face and said: "Dear Radhika, you're a sweet girl and very very lovely. I had a great time last evening, and an even better time after that. What about you?"

She had certainly enjoyed herself at the party. She had idolised Devendra for long, and had been delighted to have finally landed a small role in his first movie as a director. The production team had organised a small celebratory party at Devendra's father's studio last night before they all left for the first outdoor location shooting schedule of the film. The party had been a blast – made more enjoyable by the fact that the young director had taken a liking for her and had stuck by her all evening.

High on drinks and drugs, she had willingly accompanied him to the hotel. The first kiss had just happened. And then the second kiss. When Devendra pressed his lips to her mouth, he found that her lips were warm and trembling. Slowly the trembling stopped and nothing but the warmth remained.

Her body was like a fire and in a moment they were in a world all of their own, on a cloud racing across the night sky. A comet caught her in its grip and then burst inside her like a shooting star. There was a startling moment of stillness and then she was tumbling into a bottomless void, completely and absolutely and irrevocably lost...

Now Devendra held her hand in a firm grip. "I love you, Radhika," he said. "I won't let you go."

The wave of relief that flooded over Radhika almost drowned her. Tears of happiness welled up in her eyes. "I – I love you, too, Devendra, love you very much!"

She could feel the muscles of her body straining with a terrible beat. Her arms had a strange strength all their own as they reached out and pulled him to her and then she held him close, very close, to her. They kissed passionately.

Radhika had fallen headlong into her first and last love affair.

Their affair was clandestine. He wanted to keep it secret until he had established himself as a successful Bollywood director – and he had won his father's approval on the professional front. She agreed readily; she would have jumped off a cliff for him, if he had asked.

And then, eight months into the relationship, she got pregnant.

Chapter Forty Two
ATTACKED AGAIN

It was a very tired Rita Sharma who boarded the chauffeur driven Toyota SUV from near the entrance of Studio One building located in Malhar Studios complex. She had been shooting throughout the day for some test sequences of her new film 'Star Struck' and attending to script reading sessions. She had tired herself out with sustained work pressure in a deliberate attempt to keep her mind away from brooding over the strange possessive streak the various men in her life had suddenly begun displaying. As the SUV shot out of the main entrance of the studio complex, she was oblivious to the crowd of fans standing outside the building who had rushed towards her vehicle and who had been promptly kept at bay by the private security guards employed by the company that owned Malhar Studios .

Neither she nor her bodyguards accompanying her in her vehicle paid any attention to the steel grey Maruti SX4 that pulled out from between a row of parked cars from across the road near the studio complex and drove off behind their Toyota SUV. The Maruti SX4 maintained a discreet distance behind the SUV, as both vehicles progressed down the highway, the driver of the smaller vehicle ensuring that there were always a couple of cars between the stalker and the stalked.

Yes, Rita was being stalked.

The young man behind the wheel of the Maruti SX4, which he had rented under false identification, was wearing large framed sunglasses and a false moustache. His eyes were completely covered by the dark glasses. The eyes hidden by the sunglasses were jet black – and they blazed with hatred…

Dhruv Solanki gripped the steering wheel with a force that reflected the violent emotions that were churning within him. He would teach Rita Sharma a lesson she would never forget, he promised to himself as he drove. She would, of course, guess the identity of the perpetrator of what was about to happen; her fall out with Dhruv had been too recent for her to mistake her attacker to be anybody else. But that was the intent; she would not betray him again, even if it meant that she would have to live in constant fear of him...

Dhruv was possessed completely by the madness of jealously and terrible feelings of emotional betrayal.

To take revenge and assert his dominance over Rita, he had gone back to his old self; from the days when, as hatchet man for his underworld don uncle, he had executed violent acts with the ease and ice-cold precision of a seasoned thug.

Rita was already half asleep in the passenger seat of the Toyota SUV as it raced through the massive gates of the exclusive condominium complex that housed her recently purchased penthouse. The apartment was one of the many perks that had come to her with the wealth generated by her mercurially successful movie career.

How the mysterious attacker got entry into the high security condominium complex was never discovered. But the attacker did gain entry. Was the attacker a resident of the condominium? Had the attacker masqueraded as a visitor? The subsequent investigations never did find out the answers to these questions...

But first things first – the attack.

The SUV braked to a halt in front of the entrance of building C. The two security bouncers jumped out of the front left and rear right of the vehicle and one of them opened the rear left door for a sleepy eyed Rita Sharma to step out.

Rita slowly stumbled out of the Toyota SUV – and then her body jerked around suddenly with the impact of the bullet that hit her left arm.

The security bouncers and bodyguards who had been assigned by JP Mishra to protect the person of Rita Sharma were highly trained. But it took them several seconds to realize what was happening. As the sound of the second gunshot split the air, they launched themselves at the stunned actress and brought her crashing to the ground. The bullet still managed to graze past the diva's left ear before smashing into the rear side window of the Toyota SUV.

As glass pieces from the shattered window flew in every direction, the security men desperately dragged a limp Rita towards the entrance doors of the building. The guard of the building had started shouting for help and running feet could be heard converging on the spot.

The attacker fired one more shot in the direction of the actress – but the security men had been very quick with their actions. Rita had been bundled into the building as the shot was fired – and the bullet missed hitting the super star or anybody else for that matter. The bullet was later discovered embedded in a grass patch on the ground next to the entrance of the building.

In the subsequent pandemonium, nobody noticed that a little while later Dhruv Solanki, still wearing large sized sunglasses, had entered a Maruti SX4 car, which had been parked down the road from the condominium complex, and had then casually driven away, the eyes behind the dark glasses still blazing with hatred…

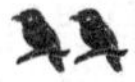

Chapter Forty Three

DESERTED BY DESTINY

Sanya and Shantanu listened in shocked silence as Radhika continued her story. Time was running out for the visitors – the jail guards would soon be telling them to leave – but they were oblivious, deeply engrossed in hearing this recounting by the prisoner of the great tragedy of her life.

"When Devendra got to know I was pregnant, he packed me off to America. He told me he could not marry me immediately; he was about to release his first film, which would make or break his career, and he could not afford distractions like marriage. He also needed time and space to explain everything to his father. I believed him completely – I was so much in love with him."

Shantanu cast a side glance at Sanya. He could guess where the story was heading…

Sanya was not a fool. "He didn't marry you, did he?"

Radhika stared down at her hands and her shoulders drooped helplessly.

Sanya was rocked by grief. There were emotions tearing at her which were numbing her senses, but she wanted to hear it all. Why and how had her mother killed her father?

"Tell me, mother, tell me everything please..."

When Radhika looked up again, her eyes were empty. She spoke tonelessly and without much life: "Your father put me up in an apartment in New York and visited me occasionally. But the frequency of his visits reduced over the months. His first film as director, the one in which I had also had a small role, had been a big success, and he was shooting two new movies simultaneously. So he had very little time to come and visit me, or so he told me. Then, when I was five months pregnant, he telephoned me and asked me to get an abortion..."

Sanya shut her eyes. Shantanu gripped her hand.

"He was insistent. He said that he could not take on the liability of a child at this stage of his career. I was stunned and confused – but I refused to abort you."

The three sat in silence for a few beats.

Then Radhika spoke – and her voice sounded lost, defeated, drowned. "Devendra told me that he would cut off all contact with me, even stop sending me money for my upkeep, if I didn't abort you. Then he cut the telephone connection – and never called again."

Shantanu looked sick. "That bastard!" he hissed.

Radhika wasn't finished. "I had one friend in Devendra's circle. This was a very talented young man called Jiten Mathur, who was being groomed by him to become a director. Devendra sent him over to me to try and convince me to change my mind regarding the abortion. He didn't succeed, of course, but, strangely, was very sympathetic and kind. He gave me some money – and told me a secret I was not supposed to know."

As Radhika paused, Shantanu said slowly: "Jiten told you that Devendra was in New York at that moment, didn't he?"

As Sanya looked at Shantanu with a strange expression in her eyes, Radhika responded slowly. "Yes, he told me that Devendra was wrapping up the last few reels of one of his new movies in New York. I was not aware of this. I was livid! I rushed to New York the next day to confront Devendra. I reached the hotel, got to know his suite number from the reception and rushed up."

Shantanu drew a deep breath. "I knew your face was a bit familiar, but I never guessed! I was exiting the lift you entered. I was leaving for the airport, my job with the patch up shots over..."

Sanya was dumbstruck. Her mouth fell open. "You – you knew my father?"

Radhika continued as if she hadn't been interrupted. "When I barged into the bedroom, there was a woman with Devendra. Both were in the bed, half clothed. Devendra jumped out of the bed when he saw me, shocked out of his wits. My blood was boiling; I was crying and screaming; I had lost all reason. I remember I shouted at him: 'You bastard! You want to kill your child so that you can screw around!' I grabbed a chair and raised it without thinking and brought it down on his head."

This time the silence was deafening.

Radhika began sobbing softly. "The chair smashed to pieces with the impact. His head split open, and there – there was blood everywhere..."

Shantanu looked as if he had been hit by a truck. He turned and stared at Sanya, who was looking at him with questions in her eyes. "Your father, Sanya, was Devendra Chopra, Brij Bhushan Chopra's only son."

Chapter Forty Four

VIOLENCE BEGETS VIOLENCE

The man did not leave the hospital until he had received confirmed news that Rita was out of danger. Then he planned his revenge.

He knew who had attacked Rita, of course. The cops were investigating, but he was ahead of them in the guessing game. The cops had found no clues; identified no suspects. But he could easily guess. Knowing well how badly Dhruv had reacted on learning about Rita's shifting loyalties, it wasn't difficult to fill in the blanks. Nobody but he had connected the dots, perhaps because nobody but he had identified in Dhruv that same streak of jealous madness which the man himself possessed in abundance. Besides, Dhruv had gone and disappeared immediately after the attack. The circumstantial evidence was damming.

The man knew where to track down Dhruv. Where else would he seek protection but from his uncle, the great don?

The man was in a terrible rage at what had been done to Rita. He had made up his mind: both uncle and nephew would pay with their lives. He planned the kills meticulously.

He stole a car. He had the car repainted. He fixed false license plates. He spent a small fortune and tapped all his contacts and bought two untraceable guns. Then he tracked down Dhruv.

The director was staying in a hotel that belonged to his uncle. The hotel was located in Goa. It stood on the main highway and faced the Arabian Sea, which was across the road.

The man packed a suitcase and drove to Goa in the stolen car.

While Rita was recovering well in the hospital in Mumbai, the man camped in Goa and kept a watch on the Raghu Basant's hotel. He was rewarded.

He saw Dhruv. He was able to study his movements.

Dhruv left the hotel only at night. He had a car to himself, a nondescript Maruti Swift. He would drive to one corner or the other of Goa for dinner and then return well past midnight. He was obviously cooling his heels in Goa, under the protection of his uncle, until the dust settled in Mumbai. He had no idea that somebody had already connected him to the attack on Rita...

The man decided to delay no further. He would have to deal with the uncle after disposing of the nephew – and then get back to Rita's side. She needed constant watch and protection. And guidance. Only *he* knew what was best for her; not even she did...

On the designated night he got into the stolen car and drove to the don's hotel. He had in the pocket of his jacket a small .22 pistol which, though it had no silencer, only gave off a sharp little 'pop'.

He had no intention of entering the hotel. The police who would arrive at the crime scene would question the staff about all the guests and those who had visited the premises that evening.

When the man arrived at the parking lot of the hotel, heavily disguised of course, he could see that the space next to Dhruv's car was vacant. He parked next to it. Then he turned off the car lights and ignition and sat in the darkness. Across the road, he saw the ocean shimmering, parted with streaks of gold that were the moonlight.

He looked at the luminous dial of his watch. It was ten o'clock.

Then the man saw Dhruv emerge from the hotel, caught in the glow of the door lights.

He waited for the director to walk over to his car. The man tensed in expectation.

Then he stared in surprise. Instead of going to his car, Dhruv walked across the road, dodging a couple of trucks. On the other side, he strolled out on to the open beach to the very edge, daring the waves. He stood there gazing at the ocean, the yellow moon hanging like a lantern on the horizon so far away. Then he turned and came back across the highway and into the parking lot. He had let the waves reach him, and there was the squish of water coming from his fashionable shoes.

The man slowly got out of his car, disguise firmly in place. The time had come.

Dhruv was almost on him. He waited for him to go past, then smiled politely to let the director get into his car. When Dhruv was inside, the man drew the gun.

Dhruv was about to put his key into the ignition, his car window down, in deference to the cool sea breeze, when he raised his eyes, aware of the shadow. At the moment the man fired, they looked into each other's eyes. Dhruv was frozen as the bullet smashed into his face, which instantly became a mask of blood, the eyes staring out. The killer yanked open the door and fired two more bullets into the top of Dhruv's head. Blood sprayed into the killer's face. Then he threw a pouch of drugs on the floor of Dhruv's car. He slammed the door shut. He ran over and hopped into his own car. He had not dropped the pistol. That would have made it look like a planned hit, instead of a drug deal gone sour.

When Dhruv was finally discovered, his face ghostly in a paler dawn, media reports centred on the fact that Dhruv was in possession of one hundred thousand rupees worth of cocaine. The death was obviously the result of a drug deal gone sour.

Only Raghu Basant knew the truth – Rita's camp had struck back.

Chapter Forty Five

MAKING AMENDS

When Jiten Mathur got Shantanu's astonishing telephone call from New York, he was in Mumbai, not in Mathura. His wife Priti was looking after the affairs of the old age home for accident victims in Mathura while Jiten himself camped in his plush apartment in Mumbai and debated whether or not to take on a new directorial venture after the great success of 'Seduction'. He was flooded with scripts – and many producers, including Brij Bhushan, were offering him small fortunes to take on their projects.

Suddenly, all this became unimportant.

The new reality he now had to grapple with was that his late friend and mentor Devendra Chopra had sired a daughter, who nobody had known about. And this daughter was none other than the beautiful and talented girl, now a big star, who Jiten had directed in 'Seduction'.

So, Radhika, the killer of Devendra, that poor unfortunate woman who had been so badly used and abused by her lover, had *lied* to Jiten when he had visited her in jail. The child was not still born!

That child had, in reality, been born living and healthy and had been spirited away by Radhika's sister to Bangalore!

This news could not be kept hidden from Brij Bhushan! It would be unforgivable!

But how to break the news? Brij Bhushan did not know that his son had a lover who was in the family way when he had died. More importantly, Brij Bhushan did not even know that his son had been killed by this lover. Brij Bhushan Chopra only knew that his son had fallen down the New York hotel stairs and broken his head and died.

Jiten Mathur, along with a few other close friends and unit members of the late young director, had conspired in a mindboggling cover up to keep the reality behind Devendra's death a secret from his family and fans and the media in India. And they had succeeded.

That cover-up had succeeded because the killer had not fled; she had surrendered to the police who had arrived at the hotel minutes after the crime. The police had been alerted by the hotel staff who had been informed of the tragedy by the woman who had been in Devendra's room when Radhika had burst in. So there had been no media frenzy regarding a manhunt for a killer. The news of the murder had got only brief inside page mention and only in a few newspapers, since the Indian film director was not known by the American public.

In less than a week, the media had never referred to the matter again.

So Jiten and the handful of film unit members present in the hotel were able to enter into a pact to protect the name and reputation of Devendra Chopra in India by hiding the truth and claiming the death to be the result of an unfortunate accident.

This had also meant keeping the father in the dark.

All these years, Jiten had strongly believed that it had been the right thing to do. Explaining the truth back in India would not have changed the reality of what Devendra had done. Explaining the truth would not have got Radhika out of Rikers Island prison. But the truth would have broken Brij Bhushan Chopra's heart, already very badly bruised by his son's unexpected death, and would have destroyed the memory of the talented director in the minds of the public. The reputation of the upcoming production house BB Chopra Productions would also have been shattered forever.

Jiten's sense of loyalty had made him push for a cover up.

But now things had changed. It would be criminal to keep daughter and grandfather apart…

Jiten Mathur stuck to form; whenever he was plagued by doubt he turned to his wife of fifteen years for counsel. He did the same now; he called Priti.

She listened to the one sided telephone call in silence. Jiten had a disturbing story to tell; she allowed him to pour it all out uninterrupted.

Then she spoke – and Jiten already knew what she would advise. "You must tell Brij ji everything. Sanya now knows that she is Devendra's daughter. So does Shantanu. So do you – and me. How can Brij ji be now kept in the dark?

There was no way Jiten could contradict that.

"Who else are in the know of the cover up?" asked Priti.

"Not Shantanu," replied Jiten. "He had left for the airport to return to India minutes before Devendra was killed. He got the news of the death only on return to India. There were two unit members present in the hotel when all this happened; the cinematographer and the script writer. We were in new York for the patch up shots of the completed film – so only the most essential crew members had gone on this trip."

"What about the woman who was in bed with Devendra, when Sanya's mother had barged into the room? Was she also in the know of the cover up? Where is she now?"

Jiten smiled grimly to himself. "She was in the know all right. She was the prime witness against Radhika, of course. She had seen the tragedy enacted in front of her eyes. But she sympathised with Radhika when she got to know the facts of the case – not that the facts helped mitigate Radhika's case with the American courts. And she went along with the cover up in India, for the sake of the reputation of Brij ji and his production house."

"She was Devendra's current lover, at that time?"

"That's why she was in bed with Devendra."

"Of course! That was a stupid question! Any idea where she is now?"

Jiten drew a deep breath. "Yes, Priti. I know where to find her. We're talking of Brij ji's secretary, Deepali Gadgil..."

Chapter Forty Six

VENGEANCE

The day Raghu Basant died was the day he had set up a meeting with a couple of friendly Mumbai underworld leaders, who were also his business associates, to plan his revenge against the superstar Rita Sharma and her billionaire protector JP Mishra. He was burning with impatience to avenge the murder of his nephew Dhruv Solanki.

Dhruv had tried to kill Rita. He had been promptly shot to death. Rita and her supporters would not get away with Dhruv's murder, Raghu promised to himself, beside himself with rage.

In spite of his anger at his nephew's murder, he also felt a frisson of excitement at the thought of the impending bloodshed…

The Mumbai sun was already a bright yellow ball in the sky when Raghu set out for his last drive.

His chauffeur driven Toyota SUV stopped at a red light traffic signal. Unnoticed by either the driver or the bodyguard in the front seats, or by Raghu Basant sitting in the back, the helmeted and sunglasses wearing motorcyclist who drove up and stopped next to the vehicle quickly reached out and stuck a metal object on the rear of the SUV, right next to the fuel tank.

The man was satisfied. He had personally ensured that the operation would not fail, though he had done so at considerable risk to himself.

The metal object was a compact, button operated bomb with a magnetic base. It stuck to the metallic surface of the vehicle like a leech. The bomb was packed with high quality explosive. It had an arming switch and destruct mechanism wired to explode within thirty seconds after the man had pressed the switch to arm the device before sticking it onto the SUV.

The minute the red light turned to amber, the man sped away. As the motorcycle disappeared, the light turned green and the driver threw the SUV into gear.

The bomb then exploded, with an ear-shattering bang! The noise was heard up to several miles away. The SUV burst into flames and was torn apart by the powerful explosion. Windows of several nearby cars shattered and there was chaos on the road. The strategic placement of the bomb right next to the fuel tank had been devastatingly effective. The vehicle had turned instantaneously into a blazing inferno.

Raghu Basant, his driver and bodyguard all died in the blast. Not much was left of them when the charred bodies were finally pulled out of the debris of the burnt out shell of the SUV.

The assassination, however, did not go all according to plan. The assassin was not able to vanish from the scene. The man could not manage to get far enough from the exploding SUV. A truck had suddenly and unexpectedly loomed up in front of the biker and blocked his escape route. The man was caught in the impact of the blast and flung from his motorcycle. He landed on the hard road with a thud and blacked out.

The man had been carrying another magnet bomb as back up – in case the first one fell while he tried to stick it on the SUV. This was his undoing. The magnet bomb was found on his person after the unconscious biker was taken to the nearest hospital.

The sensational news of the killings of Raghu Basant and his men and the capture of the bomber was overshadowed by the discovery of the identity of the murderer. It was the famous film producer Yash Kapoor.

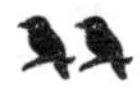

Chapter Forty Seven

GATHERING EVIDENCE AND RECOLLECTING EVENTS

Jiten had told his wife what all he would need with him when he met Brij Bhushan Chopra to tell him about his newly found grand-daughter.

Priti had been very surprised; she had never known that Jiten had such things in his custody, hidden away from her.

"How did these things come into your possession?" she asked her husband in wonder.

"I had gone to meet Radhika in prison once after her conviction," Jiten told Priti over the phone. "I knew her from before; I had met her on a couple of occasions when she was with Devendra. Then, again, I had met her in New York, on Devendra's request, to pass on his message to her to re-consider her stand on the abortion…"

"You asked Radhika to abort the child?" asked a shocked Priti.

"I've regretted it ever since," replied Jiten unhappily. "At that time, I was only passing on my dear friend's request once again to his girlfriend…"

"Radhika refused?"

"Yes. And I did not pursue the matter. In fact, I was very sorry for her, and gave her some money on an impulse to help her out. I also told her that Devendra was in New York. If I had only kept my mouth shut, the tragedy would have been averted!"

Priti was instantly comforting. "Don't say such things, Jiten! You could never have imagined that Radhika would go and kill Devendra. You were only trying to help her – giving her a chance to confront her lover in person!"

"I know, I know. That was the intent. But look what happened!"

"This is pointless, Jiten. It makes no sense to talk like this, now, after all these years. Let's focus on how we can set things right for Sanya and Brij. The circumstances that led to Devendra's death were created by him; he used and discarded Radhika; he refused to take responsibility for his child. He's no longer important. Sanya and Radhika and Brij ji are the ones who matter – we must try and make things right for them!"

As usual, it was Priti who put everything in perspective for Jiten. He drew a deep breath and said: "You're right my love – absolutely. So let's focus on the things I need you to bring quickly to Mumbai..."

When Jiten had visited her in prison after her conviction, Radhika had falsely told him that the child had been born dead. She had also had handed over to Jiten, for safe keeping, her photo albums. These were full of photographs of Devendra and her in happier times. She had also handed over her collection of letters from Devendra, which Jiten had never opened.

Jiten had also, on an impulse he did not understand then but appreciated now, kept a file of newspaper cuttings about the reports on the killing and the background of those involved. Radhika's love affair with her victim and her pregnancy had been reported in the small news items.

Priti recovered all these from the places they had been hidden by Jiten in their house in Mathura, all the while marvelling at how little she had known of this aspect of her husband's past and at his ability to keep secrets hidden from her.

Shantanu and Sanya returned to India carrying copies of prison records of Radhika's case and her delivery in the jail hospital two decades ago.

Sanya burned for justice. She wanted her mother out of Rikers Island Prison – and she wanted the full force of Brij Bhushan's power behind this effort.

While the Hindi film industry grappled with the terrible incidents involving Rita, Dhruv and Yash, and the Mumbai underworld tried to adjust to the loss of one its kingpins, Jiten, Shantanu and Deepali together met a stunned Brij Bhushan Chopra in his estate in Karjat...

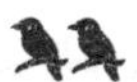

Chapter Forty Eight

THE KILLER

Rita met Yash just once after he was captured. She went to meet him in the Arthur Road Jail hospital, where he was recovering from his injuries, under heavy guard. Everybody advised her not to go; the man was clearly mad, obsessed, a dangerous psychopath – and very unpredictable. But Rita felt the need to meet him and understand.

The man was lying in his hospital bed, heavily bandaged. He had suffered serious burns from the explosion and broken many bones from the fall. But he had regained consciousness and could talk. He had confessed all to the police officials who had questioned him, but Rita still wanted a first-hand account.

"Why? Why did you do these things, Yash?"

Rita was standing next to the hospital bed, a policeman by her side and a bodyguard near the door, ready to spring to her defence at the slightest sign of danger. Considering that Yash was bandaged from head to toe and hooked up to a drip, immediate danger from him seemed a bit improbable, but you never knew with psychopaths…

Yash smiled weakly and replied: "I love you, Rita, I always have, I always will. Nobody can harm you while I am around."

"You – you killed Dhruv?"

"He tried to kill you. He was obsessed with you; he hated the thought of losing you to anybody else. He would have tried again to harm you. He had to be stopped."

Rita shut her eyes briefly. Strong emotions rocked her.

Yash continued weakly but resolutely. He was finally in a position to pour his heart out to Rita – so he did. "Raghu was also a great danger to you, Rita. He tried to kill you once before, in Delhi. I broke his knee, then, but he did not learn his lesson. So I had to finish him off. Nobody can harm you while I am around – you are too precious to me."

Rita was too shocked to say anything further. She slowly began to back away from the bed.

Yash tried to sit up and the nurse who had been standing in one corner of the room rushed forward. Yash had a maniac look in his eyes and he ignored the nurse's restraining hand. "Don't go, Rita!" he said hoarsely. "Don't leave me!"

The bodyguard pulled open the door and ushered a frightened Rita out of the room, as a couple of more nurses rushed in.

Rita was pale as she exited the room in which the director was confined – and then her face turned to parchment as she saw Yash Kapoor's wife sitting on a bench in the hospital corridor. Gayatri Kapoor's eyes were red and puffed and she had a dazed look. Rita slowly walked up to the bench and sat down beside her.

They sat in silence for a while, and then Gayatri began to weep. Rita put her arm around the devastated woman's shoulder. "I – I am sorry, Gayatri. Truly sorry. I – I had no idea..."

The other woman kept sobbing. Rita said nothing further. Disaster of unimaginable proportions had suddenly visited this unfortunate woman and her children. Their lives had so suddenly been destroyed by the madman and psychopath who had been living in their midst as husband, father, provider. There was no way anybody would ever be able to understand or share their grief...

Chapter Forty Nine

BLOODLINE

The next time Sanya Kaushik returned to Rikers Island prison complex in Queens in New York City, she had her grandfather for company.

The old man who boarded the private bus shuttle with Sanya to cross over the 1.3 kilometre Francis Buono Bridge, which straddles the East River, to go to the main prison complex from the parking lot in the south end, no longer carried his customary arrogance on his sleeve. He was a much subdued man. He had learnt that most of his adult life he had lived with a lie; his son had been killed, not died in an accident. His son had, indeed, been a genius – but a terribly flawed genius. He had a grand-daughter he had now met only when she was all grown up. And her mother was serving a life sentence for having killed his son.

Brij Bhushan had come to America to meet his grand-daughter's mother.

Radhika Kaushik was seated at her customary table in a corner of the visitors' hall, her face in the shadows. Sanya and Brij Bhushan approached her with mixed feelings. Sanya was elated that the truth was now known to her grandfather. She was hopeful that *something* would get done to get her mother out of this living hell. What that something was, she had no clue, but with Brij Bhushan's clout now having been thrown into the mix, anything was possible…

The old man had different emotions. He was going to meet his son's killer, the woman Devendra had used and abused. And with him was the daughter his son had never wanted to be born.

It was a difficult meeting. Radhika did not speak at all. Her head was kept lowered throughout the meeting and she concentrated her eyes on her hands, which were kept folded on her lap. An exasperated Sanya was beside herself with worry. "Haven't you understood, mother? Brij ji *knows!* He is formally adopting me as his daughter. The legal formalities have started for this. He is going to hire the best American lawyers to get you out of jail. You were provoked into killing dad! There are several technical grounds on which a case can be made to get you out of prison, now that you've served so many years behind bars."

Finally, Radhika raised her tired eyes, looked at both her visitors one by one and said softly, in a quavering voice: "I do not want to get out of here. I do not want to cloud your future, Sanya, with the baggage of my life. I do not want you to tell the world about me. I am glad Brij ji is adopting you as his daughter. This is as it should be. I now know that Devendra's death has been shown as an accident in India. That should not change. Let him be remembered for his films, not because of what happened to me."

Brij Bhushan cleared his throat. He was deeply troubled. "We will concentrate on getting you out of jail, first, and then think of other things. But – but you cannot suffer like this any longer. The past cannot be recovered, but you have several decades of life ahead of you – those should be better than the life you have led for the last twenty years."

Radhika had lowered her head again. She did not speak. Brij Bhushan and Sanya looked at each other with a mix of anxiety and exasperation.

When the guards asked the visitors to leave at the end of the allotted time, Radhika had still not spoken further, nor had she looked at her daughter or Brij Bhushan again, even as they kept talking to her, trying to get through and elicit responses, without much success. Their words had, apparently, fallen on deaf ears…

Chapter Fifty

END OF A CHAPTER

The prison guard at Rikers Island could never properly explain exactly how it happened. Not even after appearing before several enquiry teams.

One moment the prisoner was walking, rather shuffling, along quietly and composedly in the courtyard during the afternoon exercise hour – and then she had suddenly jumped on him with the ferociousness of a hungry tigress.

She was an old prisoner; she had been around for two decades and a little bit more. She had never given any trouble, even though she was a convicted murderer. She was thin and not very tall, her closely cropped hair giving her head the usual skull-like appearance of all prisoners. She was certainly not a person who would be expected to exhibit superhuman strength and agility. But, then, she had displayed startling power when she had smashed a chair on her victim's head two decades ago, everybody suddenly remembered…

Extreme passion can generate brief bursts of great energy, sufficient to do the necessary deed.

Radhika had pounced on the prison guard during exercise hour when his attention was briefly diverted by the antics of another prisoner at another end of the courtyard. One minute the gun was in the guard's holster, the next minute it was in her hand and the guard was on the ground, pushed off his feet by what had felt like an avalanche.

A sudden hush descended in the courtyard and other guards standing nearby swiftly drew out their guns and pointed them at the offending prisoner. Radhika pre-empted them by pointing the gun she had snatched, unwaveringly at the hapless guard lying on the ground in front of her, who was now unarmed.

The other guards did not press their triggers, though they burned to do so. They waited for Radhika's next move, desperately hoping she would not shoot their colleague. They had no intention of provoking her.

For about thirty very tense seconds the woman kept pointing the gun straight at the fallen guard. Low down, dead centre, on a line between his groin and his navel. All kinds of necessary stuff were in that region. Organs, spine, intestines, various arteries and veins. The gun was a Ruger Speed-Six. A big old .357 Magnum revolver with a short four-inch barrel, capable of blowing a hole in the guard big enough to see daylight through.

One moment the gun barrel was pointed at the guard's centre mass. Then it moved vertical. For a split second the guard on the ground thought the woman was surrendering. But the barrel kept on moving. The woman raised her chin high, like a proud, obstinate gesture. She tucked the muzzle into the soft flesh beneath it. Squeezed the trigger halfway. The cylinder turned and the hammer scraped back across the cotton of her prison uniform.

Then Radhika Kaushik pulled the trigger the rest of the way and blew her own head off.

Chapter Fifty One

GODDESSES

Sanya, Shantanu, Jiten and Brij Bhushan met Rita in her apartment. Rita had recovered, with some difficulty, from the trauma of the terrible incidents that had been linked to her. JP Mishra and Biswajeet had both been constantly by her side during the traumatic days and weeks that had followed Dhruv's and Raghu's killings and Yash's conviction.

She had immersed herself in her third film project, which was being helmed by the veteran director Dheeraj Chauhan under the banner of BB Chopra Productions, and which co-starred Biswajeet. She had studiously avoided the media under expert advice and also because she did not want to discuss Dhruv and Yash's obsession for her and Raghu's enmity with her, with anybody, much less with reporters.

What she did want to know was whether Sanya had known of Raghu's attempt on her life in Gurgaon's Ambience Mall and his further plans to harm her.

She had also learnt, to her great surprise, of Sanya's adoption by Brij Bhushan but she did not know of the blood relationship between these two, because nobody had told her of this.

So when Sanya, sounding very disturbed, had telephoned Rita and personally apologized for getting her car vandalized over a year ago, Rita did not know how to react. When Sanya told her during the same conversation that she had no clue of Raghu's violent plans towards her, Rita did not know what to believe.

Then Sanya said something very startling: "I want to meet you and tell you about my mother."

Rita was wary. She had stopped trusting Sanya a long time ago. "Why do you want to talk to me about your mother? Do I know her?"

"You don't know her, Rita. Nor will you ever get a chance to meet her now. She was in jail in America. She shot herself to death a few weeks ago."

A floodgate of shock opened up. "What – what are you saying? Jail? Shot? What is all this?" Rita paused as she heard a loud sob at the other end of the telephone connection. "I'm – I'm sorry, Sanya! This is terrible!"

The meeting took place the same day. Jiten and Shantanu took turns to fill in Rita with the story of Radhika, Devendra, Sanya, Deepali and Brij Bhushan.

"Oh, my God!" Rita had immediately reached out to Sanya and hugged her. "You poor poor girl! What a terrible time you've had!"

Then Brij Bhushan spoke. "And what a terrible life Radhika had! I – I can't believe that my son did this to her."

There was a silence as all sat immersed in their thoughts and memories. Then Sanya spoke, her eyes filled with unshed tears. "I want you to help me keep my mother's memory alive, Rita."

Rita's face was a question mark.

Brij Bhushan took over. "I want to produce a film on the story of Radhika's life. It will be a dramatisation, of course. The public and media will not know that the story of the film is based on the life of a real person. Radhika wanted to preserve Devendra's memory in the public mind as a talented film maker, and so it will remain. Jiten, who knew her, will direct it. Sanya feels that you are best suited to portray her mother..."

"You have a dramatic flair, Rita, which I do not," intervened Sanya. "You are a better actress than me. You will do justice to mother."

Rita was overwhelmed, by the story she had just heard, by the compliment, and by the proposal. She took ten seconds to decide. "I will do it," she said.

Epilogue

Nobody can go back and make a new beginning. But you can, if you want, start today, and make a new ending.

Unless, of course, you are, like me, a prisoner on death row.

Rita and Sanya made a new beginning in their relationship. Gone was the distrust and rivalry. Rita's portrayal, in a double role, of both a fictitious Radhika and a fictitious Sanya, wowed the public and the critics alike and made Brij Bhushan's movie 'A Life' a box office success of unprecedented proportions. At least this is what I have been told by my guards.

Radhika's unfortunate life has been captured for posterity on film, albeit in a fictitious avatar, as Sanya and Brij Bhushan had wanted.

I will end my story here. What happens next will be a new chapter in the lives of other people; I will no longer be a part of that drama. Will Rita continue her romance with Biswajeet? Will JP Mishra succeed in winning her heart? Will Sanya and Shantanu find everlasting happiness with each other? Is there such a thing as everlasting happiness?

As I recollect those eventful years when Rita and Sanya entered the film industry and made their mark in such dramatic fashion, I realise that I *did* have an important role to play in their history. I am glad I recorded my part in their story in the book I have managed to pen. After all, *I* was the one who gave Rita her first break, *I* was the one who protected her from Dhruv's madness, and it was *I* who saved both Rita and Sanya from Raghu's vengeance. Perhaps that was the role fate had cast me for...

My head begins to throb and I decide to stop thinking any more. In any case, my time will soon be up; my appeals for commuting of my death sentence have been rejected time and time again, and finally for one last time. I can smell death now, taste it, feel it, know it – as all my victims have known through me. Death haunts me now – and, of course, I am constantly haunted by the thought of Rita's beauty...

I love you, Rita. Live well.

THE END

OTHER BOOKS BY JOYGOPAL PODDER

Crime, Mystery and Thrillers
DECEIVERS
THE INHERITANCE
MILLENNIUM CITY
HIGH ALERT
A MILLION SECONDS TOO LATE
VANISHED

Drama, Crime and Mystery
SUPERSTAR
MUMBAI DREAMS
BEWARE OF THE NIGHT
MERCHANTS OF DREAMS

Teenage Detective Fiction
THE LANDLORD'S SECRET AND OTHER STORIES

Non-Fiction
TRUTH IS STRANGER THAN FICTION

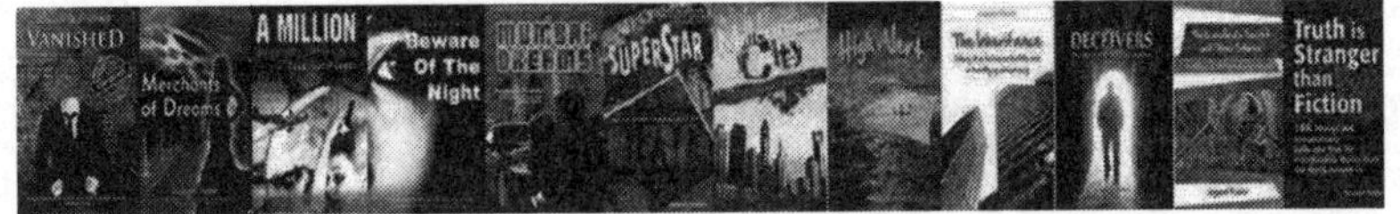